Diagnosis and Management
of Hepatic Encephalopathy

D1743686

Jasmohan S. Bajaj
Editor

Diagnosis and Management of Hepatic Encephalopathy

A Case-based Guide

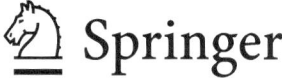 Springer

Editor
Jasmohan S. Bajaj, MBBS, MD, MS, AGAF, FAASLD, FRCP
McGuire VA Medical Center
Virginia Commonwealth University
Richmond, Virginia
USA

ISBN 978-3-319-76797-0   ISBN 978-3-319-76798-7   (eBook)
https://doi.org/10.1007/978-3-319-76798-7

Library of Congress Control Number: 2018942352

Printed on acid-free paper

This Springer imprint is published by the registered company Springer International Publishing AG part of Springer Nature
The registered company address is: Gewerbestrasse 11, 6330 Cham, Switzerland

Preface

Hepatic encephalopathy has been described extensively in the literature dating from the Egyptians to Hippocrates. The suffering of the affected patients and their companions has been a source of concern for clinicians for several centuries. With the increasing burden of liver disease worldwide, the impact of hepatic encephalopathy has only increased in both objective and subjective terms.

A multinational effort into the creation and development of key concepts in hepatic encephalopathy has culminated in the creation of ISHEN (International Society for Hepatic Encephalopathy and Nitrogen Metabolism). As its current President, I am honored to present this case-based guide on hepatic encephalopathy. The cases and chapters included here focus on the translational and clinical aspects of the evolution of hepatic encephalopathy from its minimal or covert form all the way through the end stage of liver disease. The chapters, written by some of the leading experts in hepatic encephalopathy across the world, represent a sincere effort to capture one of the most important challenges facing patients, caregivers, and clinicians that deal with chronic liver disease.

Despite this burgeoning knowledge about hepatic encephalopathy, several aspects of this fascinating disorder remain under-investigated. It is my sincere hope that this book will serve as a useful companion to clinicians as well as clinical and translational researchers who are focused on chronic liver disease and hepatic encephalopathy.

Richmond, VA, USA   Jasmohan S. Bajaj

Acknowledgments

This book is dedicated to several individuals who have helped me through the years and have focused my vision on what is important in life, clinical practice and research.

The role of my family—my mother, Amrinder Bajaj, my father, the late Chandermohan Singh Bajaj, and my brother, Deep—cannot be overstated. My pillar of support, Steven, remains steadfast, patient, and understanding in his commitment.

My mentors over the years have taught me a lot about being good clinicians, researchers, and human beings. Among the many people who have guided me are Dr. Shiv Sarin, Dr. Arun Sanyal, Dr. Patrick Kamath, Dr. Kia Saeian, and Dr. Kulwinder Dua, all of whom continue to serve as an inspiration to me.

My research family has been an integral part of my productivity. I would like to thank Ms. Melanie White, Ms. Edith Gavis, Ms. Pamela Monteith, Ms. Nicole N. Jones, Ms. Debulon Bell, Dr. Dinesh Ganapathy, Dr. Muhammad Hafeez Ullah, Dr. Allyne Topaz, and Mr. Andrew Fagan for their continued hard work and dedication.

My family extends to my workplace where my colleagues have been instrumental in shaping and executing my clinical and research focus. Prominent among these are Dr. Douglas Heuman, Ms. Ho Chong Gilles, Dr. Mitchell Schubert, Dr. Leroy Thacker, and Dr. Patrick Gillevet.

I also thank my colleagues who have given their precious time to contribute towards the chapters in this book as well as Ms. Rekha Udaiyar and Mr. Andy Kwan from Springer for their help with putting this all together.

Last but not least this book is dedicated to the brave patients and families who fight the often lonely fight with chronic liver disease and hepatic encephalopathy. Their stories have inspired all of us and we hope to alleviate these burdens in whichever way possible.

Richmond, VA, USA   Jasmohan S. Bajaj

Contents

Contributors

Chathur Acharya, M.D. Division of Gastroenterology, Hepatology and Nutrition, Virginia Commonwealth University and McGuire VA Medical Center, Richmond, VA, USA

Piero Amodio, M.D. Department of Medicine, University of Padova, Padova, Italy

Jasmohan S. Bajaj, M.D., M.S. Division of Gastroenterology, Hepatology and Nutrition, Virginia Commonwealth University and McGuire VA Medical Center, Richmond, VA, USA

Julien Bissonnette, M.D. CHUM, Université de Montréal, Montréal, QC, Canada

Amanda Briseb, M.D. Division of Palliative Care and General Internal Medicine, University of Alberta, Edmonton, AB, Canada

Radha K. Dhiman, M.D.,D.M.,F.A.C.G.,F.A.A.S.L.D. Department of Hepatology, Post Graduate Institute of Medical Education and Research, Chandigarh, India

Patrick S. Kamath, M.D. Division of Gastroenterology and Hepatology, Mayo Clinic College of Medicine, Rochester, MN, USA

Mette Munk Lauridsen, M.D. Department of Gastroenterology and Hepatology, Hospital of South West Jutland, Esbjerg, Denmark

Michael D. Leise, M.D. Division of Gastroenterology and Hepatology, Mayo Clinic College of Medicine, Rochester, MN, USA

Sudhir Maharshi, M.B.B.S., D.N.B., D.M. Department of Gastroenterology, SMS Medical College, Jaipur, India

Sara Montagnese, M.D. Department of Medicine, University of Padova, Padova, Italy

Michael Ney, M.D. Division of Gastroenterology, University of Alberta, Edmonton, AB, Canada

Thoetchai (Bee) Peeraphatdit, M.D. Division of Gastroenterology and Hepatology, Mayo Clinic College of Medicine, Rochester, MN, USA

Sahaj Rathi, M.D. Department of Hepatology, Post Graduate Institute of Medical Education and Research, Chandigarh, India

Christopher F. Rose, Ph.D. CRCHUM, Université de Montreal, Montréal, QC, Canada

Barjesh Chander Sharma, M.D., D.M. Department of Gastroenterology, G.B. Pant Hospital, New Delhi, India

Debbie Shawcross Liver Sciences, School of Immunology and Microbial Sciences, Faculty of Life Sciences and Medicine, King's College London, London, SE, UK

Puneeta Tandon, M.D. Cirrhosis Care Clinic, Division of Gastroenterology, University of Alberta, Edmonton, AB, Canada

Hendrik Vilstrup, M.D. Department of Hepatology and Gastroenterology, Aarhus University, Aarhus, Denmark

Charlotte Woodhouse Liver Sciences, School of Immunology and Microbial Sciences, Faculty of Life Sciences and Medicine, King's College London, London, SE, UK

Chapter 1
Definition and Changes in Nomenclature of Hepatic Encephalopathy

Chathur Acharya and Jasmohan S. Bajaj

Definition

The definition of hepatic encephalopathy (HE) according to the AASLD/EASL guidelines is "Brain dysfunction caused by liver insufficiency and/or PSS; it manifests as a wide spectrum of neurological or psychiatric abnormalities ranging from subclinical alterations to coma" [1]. Hence, by definition the presence of a portosystemic shunt or end-stage liver disease is not necessary. This is further explained in the nomenclature of HE.

The International Society for Hepatic Encephalopathy and Nitrogen Metabolism (ISHEN) concurred with this definition in the last meeting in 2017 and no changes were advocated to it.

C. Acharya · J. S. Bajaj, M.D., M.S. (✉)
Division of Gastroenterology, Hepatology and Nutrition, Virginia Commonwealth University and McGuire VA Medical Center, Richmond, VA, USA
e-mail: chathur.acharya@vcuhealth.org;
jasmohan.bajaj@vcuhealth.org

© Springer International Publishing AG, part of Springer Nature 2018   1
J. S. Bajaj (ed.), *Diagnosis and Management of Hepatic Encephalopathy*, https://doi.org/10.1007/978-3-319-76798-7_1

Current Issues with Nomenclature of HE

Broadly, HE is broken down into overt HE (OHE) which is Grade 2 and above on the West Haven scale/criteria (WHC) [2] and covert HE (CHE) per the ISHEN classification [3]. Table 1.1 explains the overlap in more details.

From a clinician's perspective the difference between minimal and Grade 1 HE is elusive often due to subjectivity. However, Grade 1 HE or CHE is easily differentiated from OHE by the presence of asterixis and hence the classification holds value. Grade 1 HE, given its subtle nature, can be differentiated from MHE with the help of the patient's caregivers and if the clinician has a long-standing relationship with the patient. MHE by definition has no clinical manifestation, just psychometric and neurophysiological abnormalities on specialized testing. From a clinical perspective MHE has a varied clinical course from Grade 1 OHE [4] so there is an ongoing debate as to whether the term CHE should be done away with and the old classification be adopted again. From a researcher's standpoint clubbing Grade 1 HE and MHE for study purposes allows more study recruitment and helps to easily create groups.

Table 1.1 Nomenclature guide for HE components for incorporation

Based on underlying disease	Based on WHC severity scale	Based on ISHEN	Based on time course	Based on precipitating factors
A	MHE			
B	Grade 1	Covert	Episodic	Spontaneous
C	Grade 2			
	Grade3	Overt	Recurrent	Precipitated
	Grade 4		Persistent	

This was formally tested using standardized simulated patient videos across seven centers across North America for both trainees and independent practitioners. There was a significant concordance for grades 2–4 (>90%), which dropped to <60% for patients who were normal or had Grade 1 HE. This justifies the need for a covert HE diagnosis until better user-friendly techniques are developed to diagnose Grade 1 HE [5].

Classification

The current approach to the nomenclature of HE relies on four main axes. This concept was first introduced in the world gastroenterology congress in 1998 [6] and has been followed since after minor changes by ISHEN in 2011 and formally being introduced in the last HE guidelines. The consensus is that this approach encompasses all the elements relevant to HE and can aid in appropriate treatment, continuity of care, and uniformity in research models if followed universally. Each axis in itself is a subtopic and hence taken as a whole the methodology provides all the pertinent information. Table 1.1 lists the nomenclature guide.

The four axes are as follows.

1. Underlying disease:
   As mentioned in the definition, the presence of HE does not require the presence of a portosystemic or chronic liver disease for that matter and this is reflected in this axis. Based on the underlying pathology there are three types of HE:

   (a) Type A resultant of (A)cute liver failure
   (b) Type B resultant of portosystemic (B)ypass/shunting from other non-liver-related pathology
   (c) Type C resultant of (C)irrhosis

Based on these subtypes we can see that Type C is the most common form that one will clinically encounter. Phenotypically Type C will have stigmata of cirrhosis as HE manifests on decompensation but the HE manifestations will be similar to Type B. Type A which has a separate pathophysiology due to acuity of disease process clinically appears different and has a different approach to management. Knowledge of etiology guides management.

2. Severity of manifestation:

This axis is the most contentious part of the classification. This is as per the current grading of severity scale (WHC), though universally accepted as a standard, not thought to be objective and is arguably more subjective. Table 1.2 describes

Table 1.2 West Haven criteria as proposed by Conn et al. with comparison to ISHEN grading

Grade of HE on WHC	Clinical manifestation	ISHEN Grade
Minimal	No clinical features	Covert hepatic encephalopathy
Grade 1	Trivial lack of awareness Euphoria or anxiety Shortened attention span Impairment of addition or subtraction Altered sleep rhythm	
Grade 2	Lethargy or apathy Disorientation for time Obvious personality change Inappropriate behavior Dyspraxia **Asterixis**	Overt hepatic encephalopathy
Grade 3	Somnolence to semistupor Responsive to stimuli Confused Gross disorientation Bizarre behavior	
Grade 4	Coma	

this scale in detail. The second point of contention is the nomenclature of that of CHE as mentioned above. Again, though currently accepted as standard there is an ongoing debate as to the usefulness of this classification, i.e. creating an extra category of CHE and reverting to a more basic classification of minimal HE and OHE only. However, the concept of CHE was introduced to aid in attaining a more universal platform for enrolling for international clinical trials given the subjective nature of the WHC to begin with and further discussion will be done before the next consensus guidelines.

Knowledge of the severity changes our approach of medication administration and also dose of the drug. The grade also determines the location of management and can prognosticate the course [7].

3. Time course of manifestations:

The timing of HE adds to the appropriate classification as certain etiologies for precipitation are more associated with recurrent HE and some more so for episodic HE [1]. Since, these different timelines refer to obvious (overt) manifestations it is not applicable to the nomenclature of CHE. Having this information, i.e. non-HE time between episodes, helps the provider plan on long-term management strategies to alleviate the precipitating factor. Knowledge of time course also helps aid in treatment options (when to add rifaximin) and also need to recruitment for HE clinical trials (if patient can be tried on second-line medications, etc.). Figure 1.1 explains the time course of OHE.

4. Existence of precipitating factors:

There is an urgent need to look for precipitating events for OHE as correction of the underlying precipitator will help in earlier resolution of the episode. Apart from instituting standard-of-care therapy for management of HE, correcting of underlying metabolic abnormalities, infections, etc. which

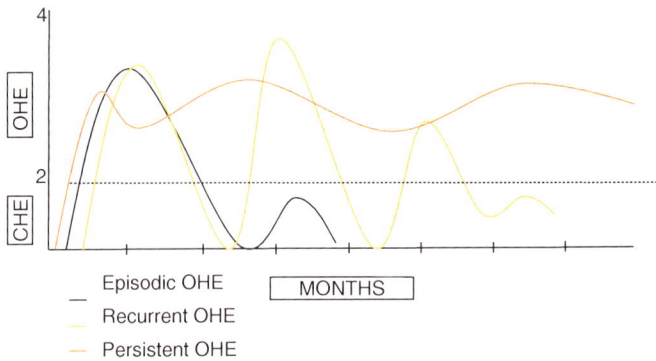

Fig. 1.1 Description of subtypes of OHE based on time course

are common precipitating factors helps. Sometimes despite extensive evaluation a precipitating factor is not found and then the episode is labelled as spontaneous.

The importance of combining all these axes into a unified description of HE is imperative for continued care of patients and also for the current provider to recognize precipitants that can be remedied to prevent the long-term consequences of HE. Knowing a patient's entire HE-related course/information lends for a strong foundation for being proactive in care.

To help the reader put this nomenclature to practice and to emphasize the importance we will provide a variety of examples.

Case 1

A 60-year-old female with hepatitis C-related cirrhosis is admitted to your hospital for the third time in a 5-month period with an episode of acute confusions diagnosed as HE. On examination the patient is noncoherent, lethargic, and disoriented to time and place, and has no focal neurological deficits but does have asterixis. No ascites or edema was noted on exam and this was confirmed on radiological studies of the abdomen. Lab work including drug screen was only notable for an acute kidney injury and elevated ammonia levels. Previous admission urinalysis was significant for UTI. She is already on lactulose and rifaximin and takes step 1 diuretics. Per caregivers she has been compliant with three to four bowel movements a day. She was continued on home meds and given IV fluids and was discharged home with changes to her diuretic regimen.

Based on the current recommendations let us examine the diagnosis.

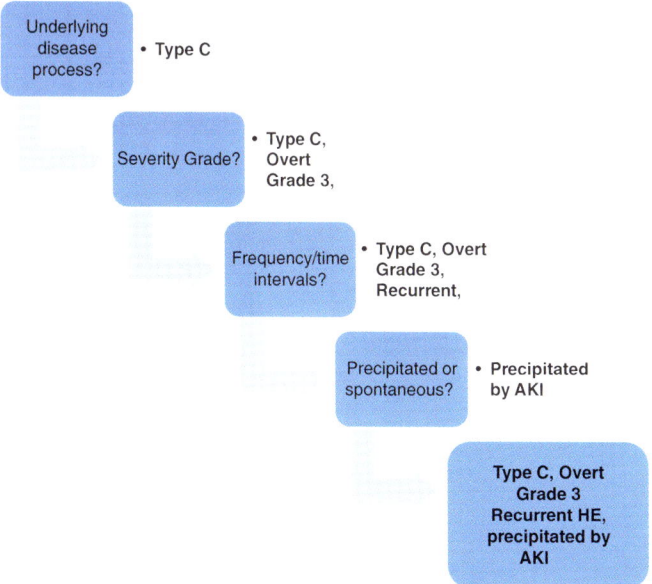

Case 2

A 46-year-old man with chronic alcoholic cirrhosis with abstinence from alcohol for the past 2 years is seen in your clinic for
complaints of episodes of confusion. The patient's daughter
who is accompanying the patient states that "Dad has been act-
ing weird" for the last couple of weeks. The patient does say
that he did get a little confused while driving to the store a week
back. On examination, there is no ascites or asterixis and the
patient is oriented to time, place, and person. Investigation does
not reveal any signs of infection and all laboratory workup
including a drug screen is within normal limits. The patient is
evaluated by the hospital's hepatic encephalopathy research
team and is found to be impaired on psychometric and neurophysiological testing.

Based on the current recommendations let us examine the
diagnosis.

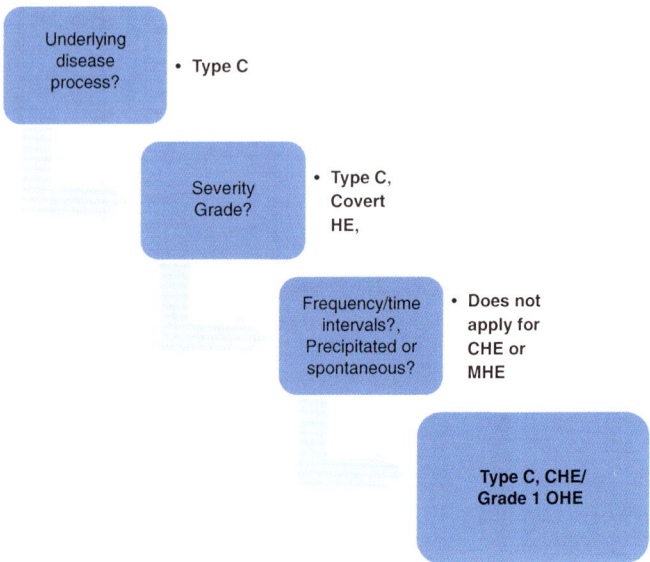

Case 3

A 48-year-old woman with obesity and nonalcoholic steato-hepatitis, with a new fibroscan diagnosis of cirrhosis, presents to your clinic for discussion of the plan of care. Review of lab work does show some hepatitis. She is employed as a ride-sharing taxi driver. On examination, there no asterixis and she is oriented to time, place, and person. She says that she has been feeling well and does not really have any complaints. Given her job and potential for neurocognitive impairment she was referred to the hepatic encephalopathy research group for neurocognitive and psychometric testing. Results were abnormal and she was advised to start an empiric trial of lactulose.

Based on the current recommendations let us examine the diagnosis.

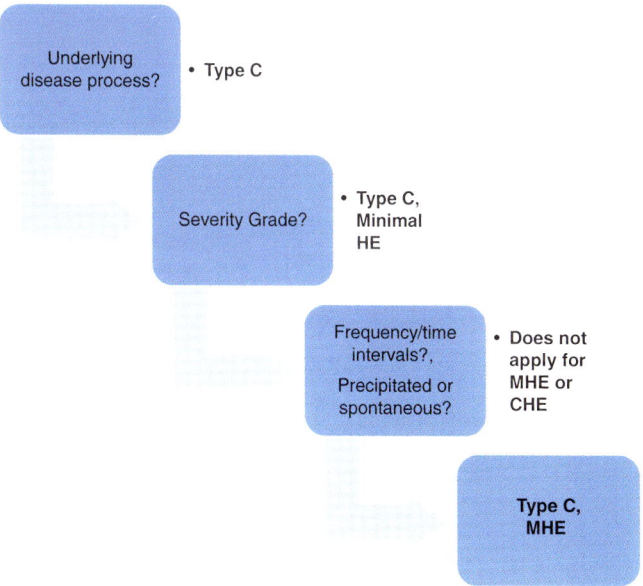

Case 4

A 58-year-old female with primary biliary cirrhosis awaiting trans-plant presents to your hospital's emergency room for acute confu-sion. Her course of recent events has been complicated by refractory ascites requiring serial large-volume paracentesis and multiple episodes of encephalopathy requiring admission. Despite optimal therapy with lactulose and rifaximin for 7 months, step 3 diuretics, she has not improved much. On presentation she feels she is at her baseline. She appears to be slow, is oriented to place, and on exam has obvious jaundice, asterixis, ascites, and edema. Her partner and caregiver report that she is taking all her medications as prescribed but still has been confused for the most part over the last 6–7 months. Labs including comprehensive metabolic panel, uri-nalysis, and toxicology screen are all within normal. Pt is admitted for management of ascites and for hepatic encephalopathy.

Based on the current recommendations let us examine the diagnosis.

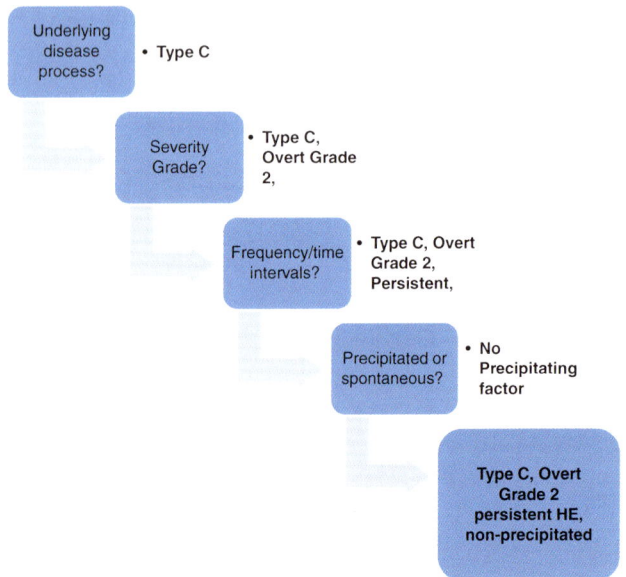

Case 5

A 38-year-old female with alcoholic cirrhosis, now abstinent for 11 months, presents to your emergency room for confusion. She appears to be hemodynamically stable and laboratory work per ER is essentially normal except for mild elevation in her liver functions and for ammonia being elevated. She is oriented to place but appears drowsy while conversing. Examination is unremarkable except for asterixis. You order a drug screen which is negative. Urinalysis and chest X-ray are negative. You admit the patient for management of HE and start her on lactulose orally.

Based on the current recommendations let us examine the diagnosis.

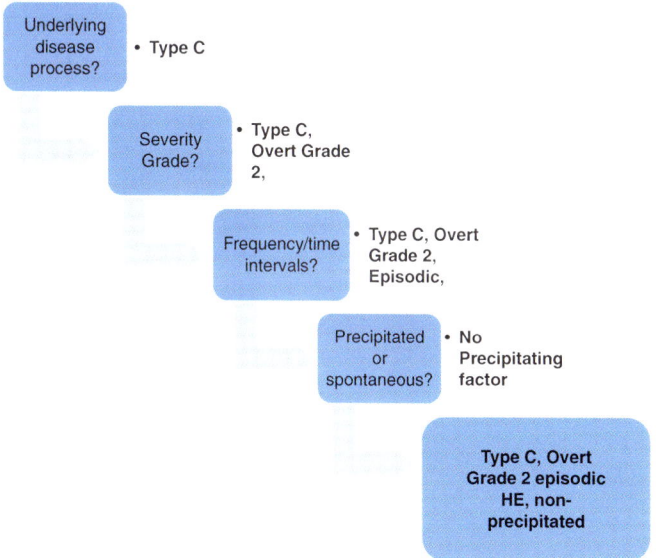

Conclusion

The definition of HE has reached a consensus and one might not see much change there over the next decade. The nomenclature of HE, on the other hand, is more complex and has many aspects that need more research and debate on. The broad components may not see much change but as our data and research progress the subcategories may evolve. As we stand, the four axes for categorizing the HE provide the appropriate information to understand the current episode and help device strategies for treatment and prevention. The main goal to help improve the quality of care for this very sick population is well met with the current system of nomenclature but further research in this field will help us refine this further.

References

1. Vilstrup H, Amodio P, Bajaj J, Cordoba J, Ferenci P, Mullen KD, Weissenborn K, Wong P. Hepatic encephalopathy in chronic liver disease: 2014 Practice Guideline by the American Association for the Study of Liver Diseases and the European Association for the Study of the Liver. Hepatology. 2014;60(2):715–35.
2. Conn HO, Leevy CM, Vlahcevic ZR, Rodgers JB, Maddrey WC, Seeff L, Levy LL. Comparison of lactulose and neomycin in the treatment of chronic portal-systemic encephalopathy. A double blind controlled trial. Gastroenterology. 1977;72(4 Pt 1):573–83.
3. Bajaj JS, Cordoba J, Mullen KD, Amodio P, Shawcross DL, Butterworth RF, Morgan MY, International Society for Hepatic Encephalopathy and Nitrogen Metabolism (ISHEN). Review article: the design of clinical trials in hepatic encephalopathy—an International Society for Hepatic Encephalopathy and Nitrogen Metabolism (ISHEN) consensus statement. Aliment Pharmacol Ther. 2011;33(7):739–47.
4. Thomsen KL, Macnaughtan J, Tritto G, Mookerjee RP, Jalan R. Clinical and pathophysiological characteristics of cirrhotic patients with grade 1 and minimal hepatic encephalopathy. PloS One. 2016;11(1):e0146076.

5. Reuter B, Walter K, Bissonette J, Leise MD, Lai J, Tandon P, Kamath PS, Biggins SW, Rose CF, Wade JB, Bajaj JS. Assessment of the spectrum of hepatic encephalopathy: a multi-center study. Liver Transpl. 2018; doi: 10.1002/lt.25032. [Epub ahead of print] PMID: 29457869
6. Ferenci P, Lockwood A, Mullen K, Tarter R, Weissenborn K, Blei AT. Hepatic encephalopathy—definition, nomenclature, diagnosis, and quantification: final report of the working party at the 11th World Congresses of Gastroenterology, Vienna, 1998. Hepatology. 2002;35(3):716–21.
7. Stewart CA, Malinchoc M, Kim WR, Kamath PS. Hepatic encephalopathy as a predictor of survival in patients with end-stage liver disease. Liver Transplant. 2007;13(10):1366–71.

Chapter 2
Hepatic Encephalopathy: Pathophysiology—Brain

Julien Bissonnette and Christopher F. Rose

Clinical Scenario

Part 1: *A 58-year-old male with nonalcoholic steatohepatitis (NASH) cirrhosis presents for routine follow-up. He has no history of decompensation of his liver disease and is currently taking furosemide to control lower limb edema. When questioned, he has no specific complaints. However, his wife reports that for the past 3 months, she has noticed changes in his behavior. She states that he is moody, often wakes up during the night (interrupting her sleep), is forgetful, and has missed a few days at work. In addition, he was recently involved in a minor car accident. She also states that her husband has lost 12 pounds over the last 6 months. Physical examination reveals an alert and oriented patient with normal vital signs, no ascites, or flapping tremor. Body mass index is at 31 kg/m2. The physician notices a clear loss of muscle mass since the last visit, including*

J. Bissonnette, M.D.
CHUM, Université de Montréal, Montréal, Québec, Canada

C. F. Rose, Ph.D. (✉)
CRCHUM, Université de Montréal, Montréal, Québec, Canada
e-mail: christopher.rose@umontreal.ca

© Springer International Publishing AG, part of Springer Nature 2018   15
J. S. Bajaj (ed.), *Diagnosis and Management of Hepatic Encephalopathy*, https://doi.org/10.1007/978-3-319-76798-7_2

temporal muscle wasting. He has no signs of gastrointestinal bleeding or infection. Blood work reveals moderate thrombocytopenia, normal hemoglobin, white blood cell count and C-reactive protein levels, preserved liver function (INR 1.2 and total bilirubin 1.9 mg/dL), and preserved kidney function. Blood level of ammonia is at 87 μM. The ultrasound reports no focal liver lesion, minimal perihepatic ascites, and a patent portal vein with a large spontaneous splenorenal shunt.

Question 1: How is the concentration of blood ammonia regulated? What are the contributing factors to hyperammonemia in chronic liver disease?

Causes of Hyperammonemia

A large amount of ammonia is generated as a by-product in the gut through the degradation of urea, protein digestion, and amino acid deamination. Subsequently, high concentrations of gut-derived ammonia are absorbed into portal venous system and filtered through the liver via the portal vein. The liver plays a vital role in regulating the circulating concentrations of ammonia (extracting 80% of ammonia) with the urea cycle (found within periportal hepatocytes) removing two molecules of ammonia for every molecule of urea produced (a high-capacity, low-affinity system). In addition, perivenous hepatocytes contain glutamine synthetase (GS), an enzyme which removes ammonia via the amination of glutamate to glutamine (a low-capacity, high-affinity system). Therefore, inevitably, a reduction in liver function leads to an increase in blood ammonia which consequently causes alterations in whole-body ammonia metabolism [1]. Alternatively, portal-systemic shunting (portal vein blood bypassing the liver) can also lead to hyperammonemia. In patients with liver disease, portosystemic collateral pathways can become significant following dilatation of preexisting anastomoses between the portal and systemic venous systems. This facilitates shunting of blood away from the liver into the systemic venous system as a means for reducing portal venous pressure (portal hypertension). In addition, hyperammonemia also frequently develops in patients with congenital portal-systemic shunting (even without any signs of liver disease) [2]. If spontaneous portosystemic shunts do not develop and portal hypertension and ascites persist, cirrhotic patients may undergo a transjugular intrahepatic portosystemic shunt (TIPS) which often leads to hyperammonemia [3]. Aside the liver, skeletal muscle, since it expresses GS [4], also has the capacity to eliminate ammonia which becomes important in regulating the circulating concentrations of ammonia during liver failure [5]. However, muscle mass loss as well as increased intramuscular adipose tissue (myosteatosis) leading to poor muscle quality weaken the capacity of muscle to clear ammonia. As a result cirrhotic patients who present with myosteatosis (due to overweight or obesity) and/or malnutrition are at a higher risk of developing hyperammonemia [6, 7].

Following the wife's observations of her husband changes in behavior, the patient undergoes the EncephalApp Stroop test with a result of 232 s (90 s with Stroop effect "off" and 142 s with Stroop effect "on"), expected result below 162 s for age, gender, and education level (based on American norms). A diagnosis of covert HE is made.

Question 2: How can ammonia explain altered mental status in this patient?

Neurotoxicity of Ammonia

Ammonia is considered an important factor in the pathogenesis of HE as hyperammonemia consequently leads to increased brain ammonia. Ammonia, at physiological pH (7.4), is primarily found (98%) in ionic form (NH_4^+), with the remaining 2% as a gas (NH_3). Ammonia, as a gas and ion, acts as a weak base and a weak acid, respectively, and therefore ammonia can accept and donate protons which denotes that changes in ammonia cause fluctuations in pH. Ammonia is quite distinct from other weak bases and acids, since NH_4^+ is very comparable in size and contains similar properties to K^+ [8]. This entails that ammonia can cross all cell membranes both as NH_3 via diffusion and as NH_4^+ via K^+ channels and transporters [9]. Therefore, due to the latter, increased concentrations of ammonia can cause shifts in cellular resting membrane [10]. Overall, throughout the body, in various organs and cell types, ammonia is produced and consumed in a number of biochemical reactions. Hence, elevated concentrations of ammonia, in addition to influencing pH and membrane potential, can also impact on cellular metabolism [11].

It is well documented that elevated levels of ammonia are toxic to the brain [12]. However, the initial effects of ammonia are not specific to the brain and it has recently been described that elevated ammonia levels can impact the function of other organs [13] (including the muscle) [14]. Nevertheless, the brain is the most sensitive organ to elevated concentrations of ammonia due to the high metabolic rate of this complex organ. A plethora of pathophysiological mechanisms and pathways have been described to underlie the neurotoxic effects of ammonia [9]. Elevated brain ammonia has been shown to disrupt neuron-neuron signaling consequently causing variations in extracellular concentration of neurotransmitters and affecting neurotransmission (glutamatergic, GABAergic, dopaminergic, serotonergic, etc.) [15]. Several lines of evidence demonstrate support for increased GABAergic tone in HE, particularly due to increased synthesis of neurosteroids in the brain which have potent positive allosteric modulatory action on the GABA-A receptor complex [16]. Neurotransmitter transporter and receptor systems have been shown to be affected by elevated ammonia, including changes in membrane expression and initiation of posttranslational protein modifications contributing to disturbed signal transduction pathways [17]. An increase in brain water has been demonstrated to be associated with HE [18] with the plausible cause due to astrocyte swelling [19]. Since the astrocyte is the sole cell within the brain that is capable of removing ammonia since it expresses GS, the accumulation of ammonia-derived glutamine within the astrocyte leading to hypertonicity is believed to be the underlying cause of astrocyte swelling. However, recent evidence suggests that lactate may also play an important role in the onset of astrocyte swelling and brain edema [20, 21]. Independent of the cause, a swollen astrocyte per se can alter astrocyte function precipitating impairment in neuron-astrocyte signaling [22]. It remains controversial on whether breakdown of the blood-brain barrier (BBB) is responsible for the development of brain edema [23]. However, an increase in BBB permeability (independent of breakdown) has been recognized as a contributing factor to the onset of HE.

The patient is prescribed lactulose at 30 mL three times daily, regularly, and is referred to a dietitian for assessment of nutritional status.

Part 2: *Two months later, the patient presents to the emergency department with fever, chills, and altered mental status with gross disorientation and slurred speech. Physical examination reveals a temperature of 38.3°C, abundant ascites, and asterixis with no lateralization of brain function on neurological examination. The wife reports that the patient has not been taking lactulose because of abdominal bloating and diarrhea. Blood work shows neutrophilia, no important deterioration of liver function (INR 1.2 and total bilirubin 2.1 mg/dL), and preserved kidney function with hyponatremia (127 mmol/L). The abdominal tap draws turbid liquid with 1800 white blood cells per mm3 (90% polymorphonuclear cells) and Gram-negative rods. Ammonia is measured at 92 μM.*

A diagnosis of spontaneous bacterial peritonitis is made, precipitating overt HE. The patient is admitted to the medical ward. He is treated with intravenous antibiotics, isotonic hydra-tion, albumin and lactulose is cautiously reintroduced.

Question 3: How does systemic inflammation/oxidative stress lead to neurologic impairment in patients with chronic liver disease?

Systemic Inflammation and Oxidative Stress

Systemic inflammation and oxidative stress have been identified as important factors in the onset of HE [24, 25]. Blood inflammatory mediators as well as markers of oxidative stress are often detected in patients with cirrhosis primarily arising from the ailing liver. Liver disease also hastens immune impairment, consequently rendering patients with cirrhosis susceptible to infection. An increase in reactive oxygen species (ROS) production from hepatocyte necrosis together with a reduction in the liver's capacity to synthesize antioxidants magnifies the induction of systemic oxidative stress. Circulating pro-inflammatory cytokines and ROS can influence the neurological function by impacting the BBB [26, 27]. The BBB, the interface between the blood and brain, is affected by ROS and inflammatory mediators as they can impact the expression of transporters and receptors along the luminal side endothelial cells lining the BBB. In turn, signaling pathways across the BBB are disturbed. Increased levels or accelerated generation of ROS, such as superoxide anion and hydroxyl radical, have been reported in the plasma of patients with liver disease [28]. ROS are highly reactive and can bind to proteins, DNA, RNA, and lipids affecting their function. Pro-inflammatory cytokines can directly pass into the brain via various transport systems and furthermore can bind with their respective receptors expressed along the cerebral endothelium causing alterations in BBB permeability [29, 30].

It has been described that "moderate" elevations of ammonia, systemic inflammation, and oxidative stress independently do not lead to HE. However, the "moderate" levels of these pathogenic factors synergistically can precipitate neurological decline. It has been demonstrated that systemic inflammation exacerbates the neuropsychological effects of hyperammonemia [31] and contributes to advanced HE [32, 33]. Similarly, in both animal and human studies, a synergistic effect of systemic oxidative stress and hyperammonemia has been shown to induce HE [25]. Plasma levels of 3-nitrotyrosine (a marker of oxidative stress) differentiated cirrhotic patients with and without minimal hepatic encephalopathy with similar degrees of hyperammonemia [34]. Bosoi et al. elegantly demonstrated that systemic oxidative stress and hyperammonemia are independent factors and that lowering either systemic oxidative stress or hyperammonemia in BDL rats leads to an attenuation in brain edema [35, 36]. In addition, inducing systemic oxidative stress in hyperammonemic portacaval shunted rats leads to the onset of brain edema [37]. A two-hit hypothesis has been proposed to be involved in the onset of HE and it has been shown that ammonia sensitizes the brain to the effects of systemic inflammation [38]; however whether the order of the pathogenic events and/or the preconditioning of a pathogenic factor has any important significance remains to be determined.

Markers of neuroinflammation and cerebral oxidative stress have also been demonstrated to be associated with HE and it is speculated that these factors may be related to HE severity. *In vitro* studies (cultured astrocytes) have demonstrated that high concentrations of ammonia (5 mM) can induce oxidative stress [39]. However, in hyperammonemic cirrhotic rats with MHE, no signs of oxidative stress in the brain [36] were observed, suggesting that lower blood ammonia levels (between 100 and 250 μM) do not stimulate cerebral oxidative stress. Furthermore, oxidative modifications of cerebral proteins and RNA as well as microglial activation were found in postmortem brain tissue from cirrhotic patients who died with overt HE [40, 41]. Nevertheless, cirrhotic rats with MHE show evidence of neuro-inflammation [42] and therefore it is speculated that nitrosative and oxidative modifications (proteins, RNA, DNA, and lipids) may be the triggering factor in the development of overt HE.

Six days later, the infection is resolved and the patient is back to his normal functioning. He is discharged home with lactulose and instructed to take the dose that will produce two to three bowel movements in a day, and ciprofloxacin as secondary prophylaxis of spontaneous bacterial peritonitis.

Part 3: *Three months later, the patient consults again at the emergency department for diarrhea that has been present for 4 days, along with fever and altered mental status. The patient has been observant to his lactulose prescription, except for the previous 24 h because of the new-onset diarrhea. Physical examination discloses hyperthermia (38.2°C), slurred speech, no gross disorientation, and flapping tremor. Abdominal tenderness is present, but with no obvious ascites.*

Blood work reveals neutrophilia, deterioration of liver function (total bilirubin at 4.7 mg/dL and INR at 1.6), and kidney function. C-reactive protein is elevated at 42 mg/L and blood ammonia at 72 μM. A stool sample is positive for the presence of Clostridium difficile antigen.

A diagnosis of Clostridium difficile colitis is made. The patient is admitted to the medical ward and treated with oral vancomycin and intravenous hydration. Ciprofloxacin prophylaxis is stopped." Eight days later, after improvement in his neurological status and clinical resolution of the infection, he is discharged home with long-term treatment with lactulose and rifaximin. Outpatient evaluation for liver transplantation is planned because of the decline in liver function.

Question 4: Is hepatic encephalopathy fully reversible or do repeated episodes of overt HE lead to permanent sequelae?

Impact of Recurrent HE

HE is defined as a metabolic disorder and therefore the brain is expected to fully recover following liver transplantation (LT). However, even following the implantation of a new liver, persisting neurological complications remain a problem affecting 8–47% of liver-transplant recipients [43–48]. Retrospective studies documented that cirrhotic patients with a history of existing bouts of overt HE were associated with impaired neurological resolution, with an increased risk of mortality and morbidity following LT [49]. In addition, pretransplant severe HE results in prolonged hospital stays post-LT which renders patients more vulnerable to nosocomial infections [49]. Persistent cognitive impairment related to learning, tested using the psychometric hepatic encephalopathy score (PHES), inhibitory control test (ICT), and EncephalApp Stroop test, has been demonstrated to occur in cirrhotic patients with preexisting bouts of OHE [50–52]. As a result, these patients are difficult to treat as they respond poorly to adequate medical therapy [53]. There is increasing evidence that recurrent HE leads to permanent cell damage. Cerebral cortical and white matter lesions have been demonstrated in patients with chronic HE [54]. Furthermore, cirrhotic patients with preexisting HE are associated with reduction in brain volume post-LT indicating signs of neuronal loss [44, 55]. Recently, an animal model of recurrent HE was characterized where episodes of overt HE were induced in portacaval shunted rats. Modulation of neurodegeneration-related genes as well as existence of neuronal cell loss in cerebellum [56] were observed to occur following multiple episodes of overt HE. Interestingly, increased mRNA expression of senescence-associated genes was found in postmortem brain samples from cirrhotic patients who died with OHE, an indication of cell cycle arrest and cell loss [57]. In addition, persistent altered mental status post-LT may lead to a reduced dose of immunosuppression (calcineurin inhibitors) and therefore may increase the risk of rejection [58]. However, in addition to pre-existing episodes of OHE possibly leading to permanent cell damage or injury, it has also been demonstrated that the strongest predictor of postoperative neurological morbidity is the presence of HE at the time of LT [43]. It is understood that the invasiveness of LT can lead to perioperative conditions that include various degrees and prolongation of anesthesia, blood loss, hypotension, and ischemia. Therefore, a compromised "frail" HE brain becomes predisposed to what would normally be an innocuous perioperative insult resulting in cell injury and death.

Conclusion

This clinical case described the importance of the interplay between hyperammonemia, systemic oxidative stress, and inflammation and their role in the development and advancement of HE. These pathogenic factors can impinge in the BBB as well as cause alterations in metabolism, cell-cell communication, and neurotransmission and lead to cognitive dysfunction. The risk of hyperammonemia rises depending on the degree of liver impairment, portal-systemic shunting, kidney function, and muscle mass quantity/quality. Liver disease increases the susceptibility of infection which can aggravate the neurotoxic effects of ammonia. It is recognized that repeated episodes of overt HE can lead to a poor prognosis, survival, as well as poor neurological outcome following LT. The latter implies that a history of HE precipitates irreversible cell injury and death. In addition, the impact of HE at the time of LT should not be neglected as a "frail" HE brain may be susceptible to minor perioperative insults occurring during surgery. While the effects of ammonia, oxidative stress, and inflammation on the brain still remain unresolved, the pathophysiological pathways underlying the continuum of HE (covert to overt to recurrent to irreversible) merit to be thoroughly investigated.

References

1. Olde Damink SWM, Deutz NEP, Dejong CHC, et al. Interorgan ammonia metabolism in liver failure. Neurochem Int. 2002;41:177–88.
2. Sokollik C, Bandsma RHJ, Gana JC, et al. Congenital portosystemic shunt: characterization of a multisystem disease. J Pediatr Gastroenterol Nutr. 2013;56:675–81. https://doi.org/10.1097/MPG.0b013e31828b3750.
3. Pereira K, Carrion AF, Martin P, et al. Current diagnosis and management of post-transjugular intrahepatic portosystemic shunt refractory hepatic encephalopathy. Liver Int. 2015;35:2487–94. https://doi.org/10.1111/liv.12956.
4. He Y, Hakvoort TBM, Vermeulen JLM, et al. Glutamine synthetase deficiency in murine astrocytes results in neonatal death. Glia. 2010;58:741–54. https://doi.org/10.1002/glia.20960.
5. Chatauret N, Desjardins P, Zwingmann C, et al. Direct molecular and spectroscopic evidence for increased ammonia removal capacity of skeletal muscle in acute liver failure. J Hepatol. 2006;44:1083–8. https://doi.org/10.1016/j.jhep.2005.11.048.
6. Merli M, Giusto M, Lucidi C, et al. Muscle depletion increases the risk of overt and minimal hepatic encephalopathy: results of a prospective study. Metab Brain Dis. 2013;28:281–4. https://doi.org/10.1007/s11011-012-9365-z.
7. Montano-Loza AJ, Angulo P, Meza-Junco J, et al. Sarcopenic obesity and myosteatosis are associated with higher mortality in patients with cirrhosis. J Cachexia Sarcopenia Muscle. 2016;7:126–35. https://doi.org/10.1002/jcsm.12039.
8. Nagaraja TN, Brookes N. Intracellular acidification induced by passive and active transport of ammonium ions in astrocytes. Am J Phys. 1998;274:C883–91.
9. Bosoi CR, Rose CF. Identifying the direct effects of ammonia on the brain. Metab Brain Dis. 2009;24:95–102. https://doi.org/10.1007/s11011-008-9112-7.

10. Allert N, Köller H, Siebler M. Ammonia-induced depolarization of cultured rat cortical astrocytes. Brain Res. 1998;782:261–70.
11. Cooper AJ, Plum F. Biochemistry and physiology of brain ammonia. Physiol Rev. 1987;67:440–519.
12. Felipo V, Butterworth RF. Neurobiology of ammonia. Prog Neurobiol. 2002;67:259–79. https://doi.org/10.1016/S0301-0082(02)00019-9.
13. Sawhney R, Holland-Fischer P, Rosselli M, et al. Role of ammonia, inflammation, and cerebral oxygenation in brain dysfunction of acute-on-chronic liver failure patients. Liver Transpl. 2016;22:732–42. https://doi.org/10.1002/lt.24443.
14. Davuluri G, Allawy A, Thapaliya S, et al. Hyperammonaemia-induced skeletal muscle mitochondrial dysfunction results in cataplerosis and oxidative stress. J Physiol. 2016;594:7341–60. https://doi.org/10.1113/JP272796.
15. Felipo V. Hepatic encephalopathy: effects of liver failure on brain function. Nat Rev Neurosci. 2013;14:851–8. https://doi.org/10.1038/nrn3587.
16. Butterworth RF. Neurosteroids in hepatic encephalopathy: novel insights and new therapeutic opportunities. J Steroid Biochem Mol Biol. 2016;160:94–7. https://doi.org/10.1016/j.jsbmb.2015.11.006.
17. Görg B, Morwinsky A, Keitel V, et al. Ammonia triggers exo-cytotic release of L-glutamate from cultured rat astrocytes. Glia. 2010a;58:691–705. https://doi.org/10.1002/glia.20955.
18. Shah NJ, Neeb H, Kircheis G, et al. Quantitative cerebral water content mapping in hepatic encephalopathy. NeuroImage. 2008;41:706–17. https://doi.org/10.1016/j.neuroimage.2008.02.057.
19. Wright G, Soper R, Brooks HF, et al. Role of aquaporin-4 in the development of brain oedema in liver failure. J Hepatol. 2010;53:91–7. https://doi.org/10.1016/j.jhep.2010.02.020.
20. Bosoi CR, Zwingmann C, Marin H, et al. Increased brain lactate is central to the development of brain edema in rats with chronic liver disease. J Hepatol. 2014b;60:554–60. https://doi.org/10.1016/j.jhep.2013.10.011.
21. Hadjihambi A, De Chiara F, Hosford PS, et al. Ammonia mediates cortical hemichannel dysfunction in rodent models of chronic liver disease. Hepatology. 2017;65:1306–18. https://doi.org/10.1002/hep.29031.
22. Sofroniew MV. Astrocyte failure as a cause of CNS dysfunction. Mol Psychiatry. 2000;5:230–2.
23. Bosoi CR, Rose CF. Brain edema in acute liver failure and chronic liver disease: similarities and differences. Neurochem Int. 2013a;62:446–57. https://doi.org/10.1016/j.neuint.2013.01.015.

24. Aldridge DR, Tranah EJ, Shawcross DL. Pathogenesis of hepatic encephalopathy: role of ammonia and systemic inflammation. J Clin Exp Hepatol. 2015;5:S7–S20. https://doi.org/10.1016/j.jceh.2014.06.004.
25. Gimenez-Garzó C, Urios A, Agustí A, et al. Is cognitive impairment in cirrhotic patients due to increased peroxynitrite and oxidative stress? Antioxid Redox Signal. 2015;22:871–7. https://doi.org/10.1089/ars.2014.6240.
26. Bosoi CR, Rose CF. Oxidative stress: a systemic factor implicated in the pathogenesis of hepatic encephalopathy. Metab Brain Dis. 2013b;28:175–8. https://doi.org/10.1007/s11011-012-9351-5.
27. Coltart I, Tranah TH, Shawcross DL. Inflammation and hepatic encephalopathy. Arch Biochem Biophys. 2013;536:189–96. https://doi.org/10.1016/j.abb.2013.03.016.
28. Chen MF, Mo LR, Lin RC, et al. Increase of resting levels of superoxide anion in the whole blood of patients with decompensated liver cirrhosis. Free Radic Biol Med. 1997;23:672–9. https://doi.org/10.1016/S0891-5849(97)00057-9.
29. de Vries HE, Blom-Roosemalen MC, van Oosten M, et al. The influence of cytokines on the integrity of the blood-brain barrier in vitro. J Neuroimmunol. 1996;64:37–43.
30. Didier N, Romero IA, Créminon C, et al. Secretion of interleukin-1beta by astrocytes mediates endothelin-1 and tumour necrosis factor-alpha effects on human brain microvascular endothelial cell permeability. J Neurochem. 2003;86:246–54.
31. Shawcross DL, Davies NA, Williams R, Jalan R. Systemic inflammatory response exacerbates the neuropsychological effects of induced hyperammonemia in cirrhosis. J Hepatol. 2004;40:247–54. https://doi.org/10.1016/j.jhep.2003.10.016.
32. Odeh M, Sabo E, Srugo I, Oliven A. Relationship between tumor necrosis factor-alpha and ammonia in patients with hepatic encephalopathy due to chronic liver failure. Ann Med. 2005;37:603–12. https://doi.org/10.1080/07853890500317414.
33. Shawcross DL, Sharifi Y, Canavan JB, et al. Infection and systemic inflammation, not ammonia, are associated with Grade 3/4 hepatic encephalopathy, but not mortality in cirrhosis. J Hepatol. 2011;54:640–9.
34. Montoliu C, Cauli O, Urios A, et al. 3-Nitro-tyrosine as a peripheral biomarker of minimal hepatic encephalopathy in patients with liver cirrhosis. Am J Gastroenterol. 2011;106:1629–37. https://doi.org/10.1038/ajg.2011.123.

35. Bosoi CR, Parent-Robitaille C, Anderson K, et al. AST-120 (spherical carbon adsorbent) lowers ammonia levels and attenuates brain edema in bile-duct ligated rats. Hepatology. 2011;53:1995–2002. https://doi.org/10.1002/hep.24273.

36. Bosoi CR, Yang X, Huynh J, et al. Systemic oxidative stress is implicated in the pathogenesis of brain edema in rats with chronic liver failure. Free Radic Biol Med. 2012;52:1228–35. https://doi.org/10.1016/j.freeradbiomed.2012.01.006.

37. Bosoi CR, Tremblay M, Rose CF. Induction of systemic oxidative stress leads to brain oedema in portacaval shunted rats. Liver Int. 2014a;34:1322–9. https://doi.org/10.1111/liv.12414.

38. Marini JC, Broussard SR. Hyperammonemia increases sensitivity to LPS. Mol Genet Metab. 2006;88:131–7. https://doi.org/10.1016/j.ymgme.2005.12.013.

39. Rama Rao KV, Jayakumar AR, Norenberg MD. Role of oxidative stress in the ammonia-induced mitochondrial permeability transition in cultured astrocytes. Neurochem Int. 2005;47:31–8. https://doi.org/10.1016/j.neuint.2005.04.004.

40. Görg B, Qvartskhava N, Bidmon H-J, et al. Oxidative stress markers in the brain of patients with cirrhosis and hepatic encephalopathy. Hepatology. 2010b;52:256–65. https://doi.org/10.1002/hep.23656.

41. Zemtsova I, Görg B, Keitel V, et al. Microglia activation in hepatic encephalopathy in rats and humans. Hepatology. 2011;54:204–15. https://doi.org/10.1002/hep.24326.

42. Rodrigo R, Cauli O, Gomez-Pinedo U, et al. Hyperammonemia induces neuroinflammation that contributes to cognitive impairment in rats with hepatic encephalopathy. Gastroenterology. 2010;139:675–84. https://doi.org/10.1053/j.gastro.2010.03.040.

43. Planas R, Ballesté B, Alvarez MA, et al. Natural history of decompensated hepatitis C virus-related cirrhosis. A study of 200 patients. J Hepatol. 2004;40:823–30. https://doi.org/10.1016/j.jhep.2004.01.005.

44. Dhar R, Young GB, Marotta P. Perioperative neurological complications after liver transplantation are best predicted by pre-transplant hepatic encephalopathy. Neurocrit Care. 2008;8:253–8. https://doi.org/10.1007/s12028-007-9020-4.

45. Sotil EU, Gottstein J, Ayala E, et al. Impact of preoperative overt hepatic encephalopathy on neurocognitive function after liver transplantation. Liver Transplant. 2009;15:184–92. https://doi.org/10.1002/lt.21593.

46. Campagna F, Biancardi A, Cillo U, et al. Neurocognitive-neurological complications of liver transplantation: a review. Metab Brain Dis. 2010;25:115–24. https://doi.org/10.1007/s11011-010-9183-0.

47. Garcia-Martinez R, Rovira A, Alonso J, et al. Hepatic encephalopathy is associated with posttransplant cognitive function and brain volume. Liver Transpl. 2011;17:38–46. https://doi.org/10.1002/lt.22197.

48. Tryc AB, Pflugrad H, Goldbecker A, et al. New-onset cognitive dysfunction impairs the quality of life in patients after liver transplantation. Liver Transpl. 2014;20:807–14. https://doi.org/10.1002/lt.23887.

49. Brandman D, Biggins SW, Hameed B, et al. Pretransplant severe hepatic encephalopathy, peritransplant sodium and post-liver transplantation morbidity and mortality. Liver Int. 2012;32:158–64. https://doi.org/10.1111/j.1478-3231.2011.02618.x.

50. Acharya C, Wade JB, Fagan A, et al. Overt hepatic encephalopathy impairs learning on the EncephalApp stroop which is reversible after liver transplantation. Liver Transpl. 2017;23:1396–403. https://doi.org/10.1002/lt.24864.

51. Bajaj JS, Schubert CM, Heuman DM, et al. Persistence of cognitive impairment after resolution of overt hepatic encephalopathy. Gastroenterology. 2010;138:2332–40. https://doi.org/10.1053/j.gastro.2010.02.015.

52. Riggio O, Ridola L, Pasquale C, et al. Evidence of persistent cognitive impairment after resolution of overt hepatic encephalopathy. Clin Gastroenterol Hepatol. 2011;9:181–3. https://doi.org/10.1016/j.cgh.2010.10.002.

53. Nardelli S, Allampati S, Riggio O, et al. Hepatic encephalopathy is associated with persistent learning impairments despite adequate medical treatment: a multicenter, international study. Dig Dis Sci. 2017;62:794–800. https://doi.org/10.1007/s10620-016-4425-6.

54. Matsusue E, Kinoshita T, Ohama E, Ogawa T. Cerebral cortical and white matter lesions in chronic hepatic encephalopathy: MR-pathologic correlations. Am J Neuroradiol. 2005;26:347–51.

55. Zeneroli ML, Cioni G, Vezzelli C, et al. Prevalence of brain atrophy in liver cirrhosis patients with chronic persistent encephalopathy: evaluation by computed tomography. J Hepatol. 1987;4:283–92.

56. García-Lezana T, Oria M, Romero-Giménez J, et al. Cerebellar neurodegeneration in a new rat model of episodic hepatic encephalopathy. J Cereb Blood Flow Metab. 2017;37:927–37. https://doi.org/10.1177/0271678X16649196.

57. Görg B, Karababa A, Shafigullina A, et al. Ammonia-induced senescence in cultured rat astrocytes and in human cerebral cortex in hepatic encephalopathy. Glia. 2015;63:37–50. https://doi.org/10.1002/glia.22731.

58. Senzolo M, Marco S, Ferronato C, et al. Neurologic complications after solid organ transplantation. Transpl Int. 2009;22:269–78. https://doi.org/10.1111/j.1432-2277.2008.00780.x.

Chapter 3
Pathophysiology: Gut Liver Axis Changes

Charlotte Woodhouse and Debbie Shawcross

Clinical Scenario: Part 1

A 65-year-old gentleman with known Child–Pugh A5 alcohol-related cirrhosis presents to the emergency department with a 24-h history of confusion. He has been abstinent from alcohol for 3 years and was stable at his last clinic review with no reported symptoms to suggest decompensation or overt neuro-cognitive dysfunction. His wife reports that since yesterday he has been agitated and disorientated and has had two episodes of melaena.

On examination, he has a Glasgow Coma Score of 14/15 and is not orientated in time or place. He has asterixis and digital rectal examination confirms melaena. There is no evidence clinically of infection or ascites but he is mildly tachycardic (110 bpm) with a blood pressure of 90/60 mmHg.

C. Woodhouse · D. Shawcross (✉)
Liver Sciences, 1st Floor JBC, School of Immunology and Microbial Sciences, Faculty of Life Sciences and Medicine, King's College London, Denmark Hill Campus, London, SE5 9RS, UK
e-mail: charlottewoodhouse@nhs.net; debbie.shawcross@kcl.ac.uk

© Springer International Publishing AG, part of Springer Nature 2018   31
J. S. Bajaj (ed.), *Diagnosis and Management of Hepatic Encephalopathy*, https://doi.org/10.1007/978-3-319-76798-7_3

Bloods on admission reveal a haemoglobin of 66 g/L with a total white cell count of 6.7×10^9 and platelets of 40,000. He has normal prothrombin time with preserved liver synthetic function and normal electrolytes.

An emergency gastroscopy undertaken following elective intubation reveals two columns of grade 2 oesophageal varices with stigmata of recent bleeding and a stomach full of dark clotted blood. There is no evidence of any active bleeding and no gastric or duodenal varices are evident. He is managed as an acute variceal bleed with oesophageal varix band ligation, transfused 2 units of packed red cells, two pools of platelets, and is extubated after 6 h as he remains cardiovascularly stable. Upon extubation he remains agitated, drowsy, and confused and is managed in the high-dependency unit. A phosphate enema twice daily is prescribed. An arterial ammonia is elevated at 140 μmol/L (normal range 12–50 μmol/L).

Ammonia

The liver and gut are intimately linked. The liver receives 75% of its blood supply directly from the gut, via the portal vein. Beneficial and toxic metabolites travel to the liver via the portal vein for processing. Traditionally, the gut has been thought of as a major site of ammonia production. Colonic bacteria produce ammonia by splitting urea and amino acids [1–3]. However, this hypothesis does not explain hyperammonaemia and HE in germ-free dogs with a portacaval shunt [4, 5], high portal-venous ammonia concentration in germ-free rats or hyperammonaemia in germ-free hepatectomized rats [6]. The alternative explanation is that hyperammonaemia arises from the intestinal breakdown of amino acids, especially glutamine. The small intestine has a high glutaminase activity, making it a major glutamine-consuming organ. Intestinal glutaminase activity is increased in cirrhosis and correlates with low-grade HE [7].

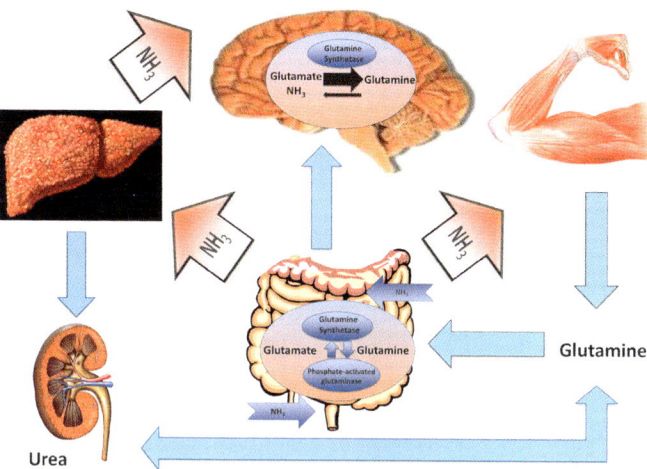

Fig. 3.1 Inter-organ ammonia and glutamine metabolism in cirrhosis

In health, ammonia is metabolised by the liver to urea, which is eliminated via the kidneys. In cirrhotic patients this pathway is attenuated owing to impaired synthetic capacity [8]. The major alternative route of ammonia detoxification is via the conversion of glutamate and ammonia to glutamine, via the action of glutamine synthetase (GS) in skeletal muscle, but astrocytes in the brain are also rich in GS (Fig. 3.1). Glutamine exerts an osmotic effect upon astrocytes, drawing water into the cell, resulting in low-grade cerebral oedema and altered mentation. This has been demonstrated by an increase in glutamine/glutamate signal using ^{1}H-magnetic resonance spectroscopy and a decrease in magnetisation transfer ratio, which is a measure of the amount of brain water. The decreased magnetisation transfer ratio correlated with worsening neuropsychological function and normalised after liver transplantation [9]. The kidney also expresses GS and can convert ammonia and glutamate into glutamine becoming an important organ for ammonia excretion. Cirrhotic patients may also have large portosystemic shunts that bypass the liver, resulting in delivery of ammonia unchanged from the gut into the systemic circulation [8].

Upper gastrointestinal bleeding in cirrhosis is associated with enhanced ammoniagenesis. Ingestion of packed red blood cells induces a significant rise in blood ammonia with the haemoglobin molecule being rich in leucine and deplete of isoleucine [10]. During a simulated upper gastrointestinal bleed in which an amino acid solution mimicking haemoglobin is given orally to patients with cirrhosis, the resulting temporary hyperammonaemia and hypoisoleucinaemia lead to a significant deterioration in memory tests, probably due to a reduction in regional cerebral perfusion [11]. This explains why acute upper gastrointestinal bleeding may be a precipitating factor for an acute episode of HE.

Clinical Scenario: Part 2

After 48 h, the patient was free of any signs of overt HE or ongoing gastrointestinal bleeding and was being managed on the ward with regular lactulose four times daily with the aim of producing at least two soft stools daily. His haemoglobin remained stable at 86 g/L. On day 3, the patient was observed by the nursing staff to once again be confused and agitated. The patient was incontinent of urine and had a low-grade fever with a temperature of 37.9 °C. There was no further evidence of ongoing gastrointestinal bleeding but a septic screen including urine and blood cultures and a chest X-ray revealed evidence of early consolidation at the right lung base and the diagnosis of a possible aspiration or ventilator-associated right lower lobe pneumonia was raised. Blood tests revealed a moderate hyponatraemia with a sodium of 130 mmol/L, an elevated leucocyte count of 14.8×10^9 and C-reactive protein of 45 IU/L (normal

<5 IU/L). The patient was commenced on broad spectrum intravenous antibiotics, given a litre of normal saline to promote renal ammonia excretion and further phosphate enemas were given.

Infection and Inflammation

Hyperammonaemia does not explain all the pathophysiological processes underpinning HE and arterial ammonia concentrations correlate poorly with clinical presentations of HE in cirrhosis [12]. The synergistic role of hyperammonaemia and infection/inflammation has been increasingly recognised [13]. Infection was shown to exacerbate neurocognitive dysfunction following an ammonia load in stable patients with cirrhosis, which resolved following antibiotic therapy [6]. Furthermore, a proinflammatory cytokine plasma milieu and not arterial ammonia or severity of liver disease per se has been shown to independently correlate with the presence and severity of HE [14]. The maintenance of a high index of suspicion of infection underlying clinical presentations of HE and expedient treatment remains pivotal in its management. Evidence also supports the administration of crystalloid to patients with stable cirrhosis as a means of promoting renal ammonia excretion [15] and is useful to deploy as a simple therapy in patients presenting with acute HE.

Clinical Scenario: Part 3

Despite 5 days of intravenous antibiotics and lactulose, the patient continued to have asterixis and had a fluctuant cognitive state with episodes of agitation and confusion worse overnight. He required one-to-one nursing. A repeat gastroscopy confirmed no evidence of any recurrent gastrointestinal bleeding and auscultation of his chest and a repeat chest X-ray suggested resolution of the pneumonia. A repeat arterial ammonia was only mildly elevated at 55 μmol/L (normal range 12–50 μmol/L). His hospital discharge was delayed by these recurrent episodes of HE graded as 2 on the West Haven Scale [16]. On day 10, now off antibiotics for 3 days, he was commenced on rifaximin in conjunction with his regular lactulose to facilitate neurocognitive recovery and to aid discharge. He was discharged from hospital on day 14 with no clinical evidence of overt HE, fully orientated in time and place.

The Gut Microbiome

The gut and liver are not only intimately linked anatomically, but also functionally, with the majority of hepatic blood flow arising from the portal vein. The portal vein carries blood directly from the bowel for processing in the liver. The liver filters metabolites of gut microbiota metabolism, as well as other beneficial products of digestion from the gut. The liver is at the forefront of the host defences against microbes. The gut wall has a variety of defences to prevent translocation of toxins from the gut lumen into the portal circulation. These include mucus produced by goblet cells, secretory IgA, bile acids and tight junctions that prevent movement of toxins between cells. Patients with cirrhosis have a more permeable gut [17], allowing translocation of endotoxin such as lipopolysaccharide (LPS, from Gram-negative cell walls) into the systemic circulation. Cirrhotic patients also have small bowel bacterial overgrowth and altered gut motility, possibly secondary to autonomic dysfunction, contributing to the overall burden of bacteria [17]. LPS binds to the pattern recognition receptor Toll-like receptor 4 (TLR4) on hepatic macrophages, causing systemic inflammation by release of pro-inflammatory cytokines [18].

In health, the gut flora is dominated by two groups of bacteria, Bacteroidetes and Firmicutes. Actinobacteria, Verrucomicrobia and Proteobacteria also contribute, but to a lesser degree [19]. Patients with cirrhosis exhibit altered bacterial composition with an overabundance of pathogenic species. A study published in 2011 showed a reduction in Bacteroidetes, with enrichment of Proteobacteria and Fusobacteria in cirrhosis. Enterobacteriaceae, Veillonellaceae and Streptococcaceae were found to be prevalent in cirrhotic patients at the family level. There was a positive relationship between Streptococcaceae and Child–Pugh score, whereas the beneficial bacteria Lachnospiriaceae were reduced in cirrhosis [20]. A second study also showed a reduction in beneficial species such as Lachnospiraceae, Ruminococcaceae and Clostridiales IV with a relative overgrowth of the potentially pathogenic Staphylococcaceae, Enterobacteriaceae and Enterococcaceae in cirrhosis. Overgrowth of Enterococcaceae may lead to endotoxaemia [21]. Dysbiosis was postulated to possibly relate to reduced bile acid synthesis in cirrhosis, along with other factors.

Cirrhotic patients with HE have a reduced relative abundance of Lachnospiriaceae and Ruminococcaceae. These species produce beneficial short-chain fatty acids (SCFAs,) which nourish colonocytes and help to lower colonic pH, thus reducing ammonia absorption. There is also an enrichment of pathogenic species such as Enterobacteriaceae [21].

A study examining the impact of synbiotics (prebiotic and probiotic in combination) on patients with minimal HE found cirrhotic patients to have an excess of pathogenic bacteria such as *E. coli* and Staphylococci [22]. This suggests that the altered microbiota in cirrhosis may play a role in the pathogenesis of HE.

Bajaj et al. noted Alcaligenaceae and Enterobacteriaceae to be differentially detected in cirrhotics with HE compared to those without HE. Alcaligenaceae (ammonia-producing species) were more abundant in those with worse cognitive performance, whereas Enterobacteriaceae correlated more with higher MELD scores and greater inflammation [23]. Enterobacteriaceae include bacteria such as *E. coli*, Shigella, Salmonella and Klebsiella, which are often the cause of infections such as spontaneous bacterial peritonitis (SBP) in cirrhotics [17].

Modifying the Gut Microbiota May Be Expected to Alter Outcomes in HE

Patients with HE have traditionally been treated with non-absorbable disaccharides such as lactulose and lactitol. Lactulose is converted to lactic and ascetic acid, acidifying the pH of the gut. This favours conversion of NH_3 to NH_4, which is less readily absorbed into the systemic circulation. The acidic milieu also discourages growth of urease-producing gut bacteria, reducing ammonia production [8, 22]. Laxatives also act as purgatives, preventing excess absorption of waste products of digestion.

Historically protein restriction had been thought to reduce nitrogenous load and hence reduce ammonia production, improving HE. A Spanish study examined the effect of protein restriction compared with normal diet on 30 patients with cirrhosis and HE. No statistically significant difference in HE outcomes was found between the two groups. Those on a low-protein diet showed higher protein catabolism. Protein restriction is consequently not recommended for patients with HE. In fact, most cirrhotic patients are malnourished with sarcopenia and protein restriction can worsen their clinical condition [24].

A systematic review by Als Nielsen et al. found insufficient evidence to recommend the use of non-absorbable disaccharides in the management of acute HE. Antibiotics such as neomycin and metronidazole were found to be superior to non-absorbable disaccharides in the management of HE, but the clinical significance of this was uncertain and their long-term use is limited by their side effects [25]. An updated systematic review published in 2016 including 38 randomised controlled trials (RCTs) enrolling 1828 participants has shown that non-absorbable disaccharides may be associated with a beneficial effect on clinically relevant outcomes compared with placebo/no intervention [26].

The non-absorbable antibiotic rifaximin has been shown to reduce recurrence of HE. A randomised, double-blind placebo-controlled trial of rifaximin in almost 300 patients with HE found that rifaximin significantly reduced the risk of an episode of HE over a 6-month period. 22.1% in the rifaximin group had breakthrough HE on rifaximin vs. 45.9% in the placebo group. Rifaximin also reduced the rate of hospitalisation for HE [27]. The majority of patients received concomitant lactulose therapy. An open-label study of patients on rifaximin for prevention of recurrent HE has shown it to have a good safety profile in follow-up of 24 months and more [28].

Rifaximin treatment improves cognition and endotoxaemia in patients with minimal HE. Fatty acid composition was altered by rifaximin therapy with increased serum-saturated and unsaturated fatty acids [29, 30]. Fatty acid changes may improve cognition [29]. No significant changes were noted in gut flora, with only a minor decrease in Veillonellaceae and increase in Eubacteriaceae [30]. Rifaximin did reduce network connectivity and clustering on the correlation networks [30]. Rifaximin may select for changes in gut microbiota that favour beneficial species, without significant changes in overall relative abundance of different species [29].

Rifaximin also favourably affects serum pro-inflammatory cytokines and faecal secondary bile acid levels [29]. Secondary bile acids such as deoxycholic acid (DCA) are associated with increased intestinal permeability, (allowing translocation of LPS into the systemic circulation) and membrane destabilisation, and alter gut flora composition. This is compounded by the fact that cirrhotic patients secrete fewer primary bile acids into the small intestine, hence promoting microbiota dysbiosis.

Rifaximin supresses faecal DCA levels [29]. Rifaximin there-fore appears to favourably alter the metabolic activity of the gut microbiota, rather than inducing huge shifts in the composition of the flora.

Modulation of gut flora seems to beneficially impact upon HE as seen by the positive impact of rifaximin and other antibi-otics on the recurrence of HE. In the era of multidrug-resistant bacteria, there is however a need to develop alternative therapies to maintain a durable response.

Modulation of the gut flora can also be achieved through use of prebiotics (food stuffs such as inulin that provide fuel to beneficial bacteria), probiotics ('healthy' bacteria such as Lactobacillus GG) and synbiotics (a combination of pre- and probiotics). A more comprehensive change in gut flora might be expected to occur if the whole dysbiotic cirrhotic gut flora were replaced with healthy bacteria. A few small studies are thus cur-rently examining the possibility of replacing the whole gut flora with faecal microbiota transplants (FMT) in humans.

A meta-analysis assessing the utility of probiotics in HE was published in 2015. The analysis looked at nine RCTs and found that probiotics were associated with an improvement in MHE and prophylaxis of overt HE. Probiotics were found to lower ammonia levels (measured in five studies only). Probiotics did not increase the rate of adverse events or mortal-ity. One hundred and thirty-five studies were identified, but only nine were deemed to be of sufficient quality for inclusion in the meta-analysis [31]. Large well-designed studies are required to confirm these findings. A more recent meta-analy-sis, published in 2016, also supported the use of probiotics in HE. This paper looked at 14 RCTs, including 1152 patients. Probiotics did not impact upon mortality and had a good safety profile. Probiotics were more effective than placebo at reduc-ing hospitalisations, improving MHE and reducing progression of MHE to overt HE; however results for probiotics were simi-lar to those seen with lactulose treatment. There was considerable heterogeneity between studies due to the use of different bacteria of varying strengths. Most studies analysed were conducted in India, so there may be dietary or environmental influences on gut flora that may not be generalisable to other populations [32].

The impact of synbiotics has also been studied in MHE. Ninety-seven cirrhotic patients with MHE, confirmed on objective testing, were treated with a synbiotic preparation, fermentable fibre alone or placebo for 30 days. An overgrowth of the potentially pathogenic species *E. coli* and Staphylococcal species was noted in cirrhosis. This was reversed with synbiotic treatment. Synbiotic treatment significantly increased the faecal content of the non-urease-producing Lactobacillus species, reducing ammonia concentrations and MHE. Synbiotics also reduced endotoxaemia. Fermentable fibre alone also improved MHE and significantly increased viable counts of the non-urease-producing Bifidobacterium spp. with an associated decrease in *E. coli* overgrowth. Fermentable fibre and synbiotics reduced colonic pH in most cases, creating an environment favouring non-urease-producing bacteria and preventing uptake of ammonia due to fermentation of the fibre to short-chain fatty acids by gut bacteria [22].

Replacing the whole dysbiotic gut flora of the cirrhotic patient with that of a healthy donor has been trialled in a handful of studies. Bajaj et al. assessed the impact of FMT in an open-label study of cirrhotic patients with recurrent HE ($n = 20$, 1:1 randomisation). FMT was administered via enema following removal of the native flora with broad-spectrum antibiotics. Five standard-of-care and no FMT participants developed further HE during the follow-up period. FMT increased diversity and beneficial taxa [33]. A Canadian case report by Kao et al. also reported improvement in HE symptoms in a patient given FMT via enema after the discontinuation of his rifaximin, but the effects of the treatment did not continue after the treatment period [34].

Conclusions

The development of overt HE in a patient with cirrhosis confers a damning prognosis with a 1-year mortality approaching 64% [35]. This complex neuropsychiatric syndrome arises as a consequence of a dysfunctional gut-liver-brain axis. Over the past 30 years, there has been a reliance on therapies aimed at lowering ammonia production or increasing metabolism following the seminal observation that the hepatic urea cycle is the major mammalian ammonia detoxification pathway and is key in the pathogenesis of HE. In cirrhosis, the relationship with ammonia is not clear-cut and it has become apparent that inflammation is a key driver and that a disrupted microbiome resulting in gut dysbiosis, bacterial overgrowth and translocation, systemic endotoxaemia and immune dysfunction may be more important drivers. Therefore, it is paramount that we aim to focus our efforts into developing therapies that modulate the disrupted microbiome or alleviating its downstream consequences.

References

1. Floch MH, Katz J, Conn HO. Qualitative and quantitative relationships of the fecal flora in cirrhotic patients with portal systemic encephalopathy and following portacaval anastomosis. Gastroenterology. 1970;59(1):70–5.
2. Weber FL Jr, Veach GL. The importance of the small intestine in gut ammonium production in the fasting dog. Gastroenterology. 1979;77(2):235–40.
3. Weber FL, Friedman DW, Fresard KM. Ammonia production from intraluminal amino acids in canine jejunum. Am J Physiol. 1988;254(2 Pt 1):G264–8.
4. Nance FC, Kaufman HJ, Kline DG. Role of urea in the hyperammonaemia of germ free Eck fistula dogs. Gastroenterology. 1974;66:108–12.
5. Kline DG, Nance FC. Eck's fistula encephalopathy in germ free dogs. Ann Surg. 1971;174(5):856–62.

6. Schalm SW, van der Mey T. Hyperammonemic coma after hepatectomy in germ-free rats. Gastroenterology. 1979;77:231–4.
7. Romero-Gomez M, Ramos-Guerrero R, Grande L, de Teran LC, Corpas R, Camacho I, et al. Intestinal glutaminase activity is increased in liver cirrhosis and correlates with minimal hepatic encephalopathy. J Hepatol. 2004;41(1):49–54.
8. Patel VC, White H, Stoy S, Bajaj JS, Shawcross DL. Clinical science workshop: targeting the gut-liver-brain axis. Metab Brain Dis. 2016;31(6):1327–37.
9. Cordoba J, Alonso J, Rovira A, Jacas C, Sanpedro F, Castells L, Vargas V, Margarit C, Kulisewsky J, Esteban R, Guardia J. The development of low-grade cerebral edema in cirrhosis is supported by the evolution of 1H-magnetic resonance abnormalities after liver transplantation. J Hepatol. 2001;35:598–604.
10. Bessman AN, Hawkins R. The relative effects of enterically administered plasma and packed cells on circulating blood ammonia. J Biol Chem. 1962;237:3151–6.
11. Jalan R, Olde Damink SWM, Lui HF, Glabus M, Deutz NEP, Hayes PC, Ebmeier K. Oral amino acid load mimicking hemoglobin results in reduced regional cerebral perfusion and deterioration in memory tests in patients with cirrhosis of the liver. Metab Brain Dis. 2003;18(1):37–49.
12. Shawcross DL, Sharifi Y, Canavan JB, Yeoman AD, Abeles RD, Taylor NJ, Auzinger G, Bernal W, Wendon JA. Infection and systemic inflammation, not ammonia, are associated with Grade 3/4 hepatic encephalopathy, but not mortality in cirrhosis. J Hepatol. 2011;54:640–9.
13. Aldridge DR, Tranah EJ, Shawcross DL. Pathogenesis of hepatic encephalopathy: role of ammonia and systemic inflammation. J Clin Exp Hepatol. 2015;5(Suppl 1):S7–S20.
14. Shawcross DL, Wright G, Olde Damink SW, Jalan R. Role of ammonia and inflammation in minimal hepatic encephalopathy. Metab Brain Dis. 2007;22(1):125–38.
15. Jalan R, Kapoor D. Enhanced renal ammonia excretion following volume expansion in patients with well compensated cirrhosis of the liver. Gut. 2003;52(7):1041–5.
16. Conn HO, Lieberthal MM. The hepatic coma syndromes and lactulose. Baltimore: Williams and Wilkins; 1979.
17. Quigley EM, Stanton C, Murphy EF. The gut microbiota and the liver. Pathophysiologcal and clinical implications. J Hepatol. 2013;58:1020–7.

18. Singh R, Bullard J, Kalra M, Assefa S, Kaul AK, Vonfeldt K, et al. Status of bacterial colonization, Toll-like receptor expression and nuclear factor-kappa B activation in normal and diseased human livers. Clin Immunol. 2011;138(1):41–9.

19. Scott KP, Gratz SW, Sheridan PO, Flint HJ, Duncan SH. The influence of diet on the gut microbiota. Pharmacol Res. 2013;69(1):52–60.

20. Chen Y, Yang F, Lu H, Wang B, Chen Y, Lei D, et al. Characterization of fecal microbial communities in patients with liver cirrhosis. Hepatology. 2011;54(2):562–72.

21. Bajaj JS, Heuman DM, Hylemin PB, Sanyal AJ, White MB. Altered profile of human gut microbiome is associated with cirrhosis and its complications. J Hepatol. 2014;60:940–7.

22. Liu Q, Duan ZP, Ha DK, Bengmark S, Kurtovic J, Riordan SM. Synbiotic modulation of gut flora: effect on minimal hepatic encephalopathy in patients with cirrhosis. Hepatology. 2004;39(5):1441–9.

23. Bajaj JS, Ridlon JM, Hylemon PB, Thacker LR, Heuman DM, Smith S, et al. Linkage of gut microbiome with cognition in hepatic encephalopathy. Am J Physiol Gastrointest Liver Physiol. 2012;302(1):G168–75.

24. Cordoba J, Lopez-Hellin J, Planas M, Sabin P, Sanpedro F, Castro F, Esteban R, Guardia J. Normal protein diet for episodic HE: results of a randomised study. J Hepatol. 2004;41:38–43.

25. Als-Nielsen B, Gluud LL, Gluud C. Non-absorbable disaccharides for hepatic encephalopathy: systematic review of randomised trials. BMJ. 2004;328(7447):1046.

26. Gluud LL, Vilstrup H, Morgan MY. Non-absorbable disaccharides versus placebo/no intervention and lactulose versus lactitol for the prevention and treatment of hepatic encephalopathy in people with cirrhosis. Cochrane Database Syst Rev. 2016;4:CD003044.

27. Bass NM, Mullen KD, Sanyal A, Poordad F, Neff G, Leevy CB. Rifaximin treatment in hepatic encephalopathy. N Engl J Med. 2010;362(12):1071–81.

28. Mullen KD, Sanyal AJ, Bass NM, Poordad FF, Sheikh MY, Frederick RT, et al. Rifaximin is safe and well tolerated for long-term maintenance of remission from overt hepatic encephalopathy. Clin Gastroenterol Hepatol. 2014;12(8):1390–7.e2.

29. Bajaj JS. Review article: potential mechanisms of action of rifaximin in the management of hepatic encephalopathy and other complications of cirrhosis. Aliment Pharmacol Ther. 2016;43(Suppl 1):11–26.

30. Bajaj JS, Heuman DM, Sanyal AJ, Hylemon PB, Sterling RK, Stravitz RT, et al. Modulation of the metabiome by rifaximin in patients

with cirrhosis and minimal hepatic encephalopathy. PLoS One. 2013;8(4):e60042.

31. Zhao LN, Yu T, Lan SY, Hou JT, Zhang ZZ, Wang SS, et al. Probiotics can improve the clinical outcomes of hepatic encephalopathy: an update meta-analysis. Clin Res Hepatol Gastroenterol. 2015;39(6):674–82.

32. Saab S, Suraweera D, Au J, Saab EG, Alper TS, Tong MJ. Probiotics are helpful in hepatic encephalopathy: a meta-analysis of randomized trials. Liver Int. 2016;36(7):986–93.

33. Bajaj JS, Kassam Z, Fagan A, Gavis EA, Liu E, Cox IJ, et al. Fecal microbiota transplant from a rational stool donor improves hepatic encephalopathy: a randomized clinical trial. Hepatology. 2017;66:1727–38.

34. Kao D, Roach B, Park H, Hotte N, Madsen K, Bain V, et al. Fecal microbiota transplantation in the management of hepatic encephalopathy. Hepatology. 2016;63(1):339–40.

35. Jepsen P, Ott P, Andersen PK, Sorensen HT, Vilstrup H. Clinical course of alcoholic liver cirrhosis: a Danish population-based cohort study. Hepatology. 2010;51(5):1675–82.

Chapter 4
Impact and Diagnosis of Minimal or Grade 1 Hepatic Encephalopathy

Mette Munk Lauridsen and Hendrik Vilstrup

Introduction

It is important to identify cirrhosis patients with minimal and grade 1 HE. They are in need of thorough information, close monitoring and well-considered treatment in order to prevent loss of quality of life, episodes of clinically manifest HE, falls and traffic accidents [1–4]. When diagnosing MHE no test strategy is more correct than the other as long as the applied tests are a measure of brain functioning and validated in the target cohort. Accordingly, several psychometric and neurophysiological tests are available for MHE diagnosis—some more thoroughly validated than others, and used in various combinations across countries and clinics depending on local resources and expertise.

_____

M. M. Lauridsen (✉)
Department of Gastroenterology and Hepatology, Hospital of South West Jutland, Esbjerg, Denmark
e-mail: mette.enok.munk.lauridsen@rsyd.dk

H. Vilstrup
Department of Hepatology and Gastroenterology, Aarhus University Hospital, Aarhus, Denmark
e-mail: vilstrup@clin.au.dk

© Springer International Publishing AG, part of Springer Nature 2018   47
J. S. Bajaj (ed.), _Diagnosis and Management of Hepatic Encephalopathy_, https://doi.org/10.1007/978-3-319-76798-7_4

Consequently, giving firm recommendations on how to diagnose minimal and grade 1 HE is difficult and not our intention. Instead we aim at illustrating how psychometric tests can be applied and interpreted regardless of the test modality. In our clinic we have a long-standing tradition for MHE testing using the continuous reaction time test (CRT), which is well validated, sensitive, fast and easy [5–11]. To encompass more cognitive functions in our evaluation of the patients, and to enable us to compare our research output with that of other clinics, we use the CRT in combination with the more widely used portosystemic encephalopathy test (PSE or PHES). In our clinic psychometric testing is conducted by a specially trained nurse and takes up 20–25 min. The purpose of the testing is not only to find patients with brain dysfunction but also to take the time to educate patient and caregivers about HE in general as most, not surprisingly, are unaware that liver disease can lead to a broad array of cerebral symptoms.

We here present two cases to demonstrate the practical use of psychometric tests and the impact of minimal and grade 1 HE on the patients' and caregivers' lives, and begin with a short introduction to the PSE and CRT test necessary to comprehend the cases.

Portosystemic Encephalopathy Test (PSE)

The PSE test is a widely used and well-validated paper-pencil psychometric test endorsed by the EASL/AASLD as a common comparator [1, 12, 13].

The PSE measures complex cognitive functions such as attention, accuracy, working speed and visual orientation. It consists of five subtests: digit symbol test, number connection test A, number connection test B, serial dotting test and line tracing test (Fig. 4.1). Completion takes 15 min for most patients. Calculating the test score from the seconds spent on each subtest takes another 5 min. If the time spent on a test is within the range of -1 to 1 standard deviation from the norm then the score given is zero. The subtest score ranges from -3 to 1. The line tracing test is evaluated by two scores—a time score and an error score. Accordingly, the summed test score, the portosystemic hepatic encephalopathy score (PHES), ranges from −18 to 6, and a result below −4 is abnormal. Language and age-adjusted norm data are available for many countries and four versions of the test battery are available to minimise learning effects at repeated testing [12, 14].

The Continuous Reaction Time Test (CRT)

The CRT is a computerised psychometric method testing the patients' ability to sustain attention for a 10-min period [9]. The patient is equipped with a set of headphones and a trigger button in the dominant hand. The computer software (EKHO, Bitmatic. com) generates sound stimuli to which the patient must react by pressing the trigger button as fast as possible. A sound stimulus is given 150 times at random intervals of 2–6 s and the main task is to stay attentive and react equally fast to each stimulus while inhibiting the urge to press the button ahead of time. The result of the test is immediately available and is given as an index (CRT index = 50 percentile/90–10 percentile) (Fig. 4.2). A CRT index below 1.9 is abnormal and indicates that the patient has unstable reaction times, i.e. might have MHE. Apart from being fast and easy to preform the CRT index has the great advantage of not being influenced by age, gender or educational level while also being able to detect improvement in brain functioning with ammonia-lowering treatment [5].

Case 1: HE with No Comorbidity

Winter 2016

A 70-year-old female with a long-standing alcohol overuse was urged by her only relatives, an adult son and daughter, to see a doctor during a period with daily vomiting and weight loss. She

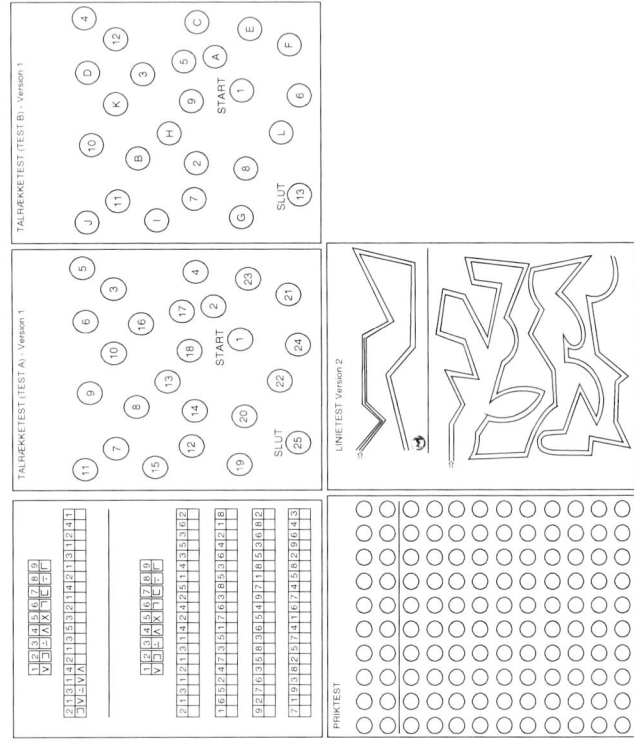

Fig. 4.1 The five paper-pencil tests of the portosystemic encephalopathy test (PSE)

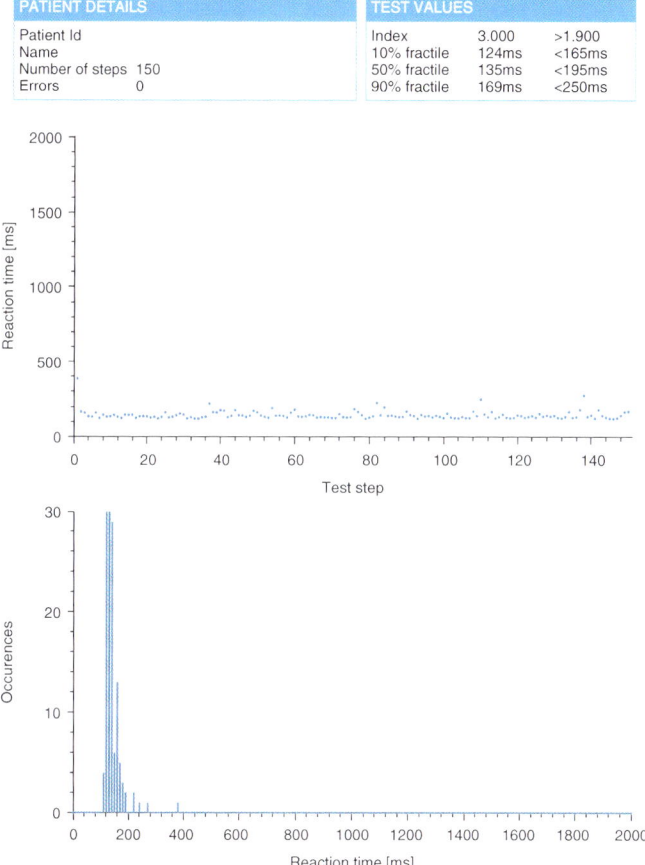

Fig. 4.2 Results from the continuous reaction time test. Panel (**a**) shows a normal result with stable reaction times, a slim distribution curve and CRT index 3.0 (below 1.9 is abnormal). Panel (**b**) shows an abnormal result with unstable reaction times, a broad distribution curve and CRT index of 0.97

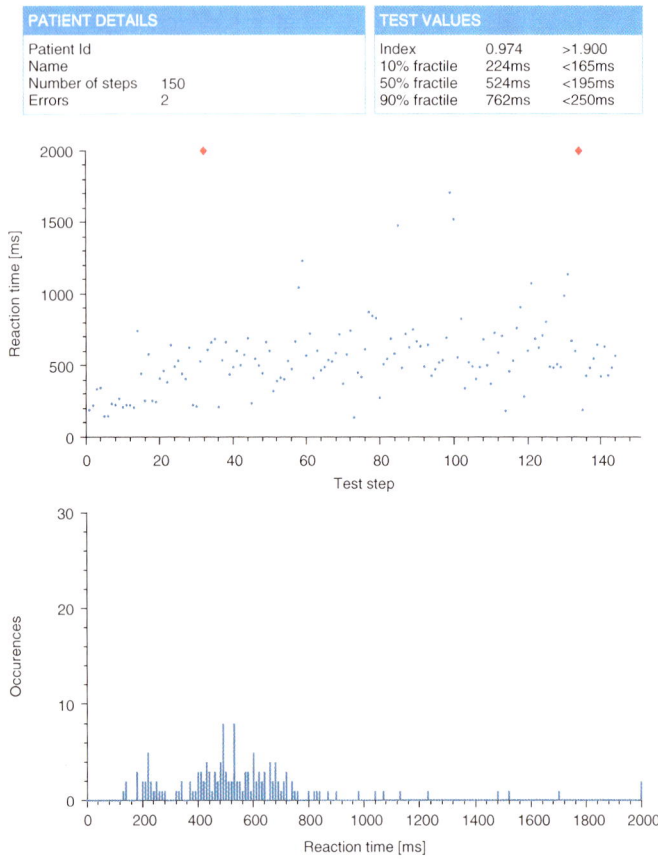

Fig. 4.2 (continued)

was referred to our clinic and we found liver cirrhosis Child-Pugh class B. At the time of diagnosis of cirrhosis the patient was malnourished, and had ascites, hyponatraemia and iron-deficiency anaemia. She stopped drinking her usual 4 units of alcohol/day at this point. There were no known co-morbidities.

The patient had been unemployed for more than 20 years and had the Danish minimum of 9 years of schooling. She had managed daily activities alone, living in an apartment in a rural area receiving state pension and getting around by car. Her son and daughter lived 40 miles away and did not maintain contact because of her long-standing alcoholism. Accordingly, she had a poor cognitive reserve [15, 16].

Treatment with diuretics was initiated and she was recommended moderate fluid restriction to mobilise ascites and correct hyponatraemia. Nutritional therapy was initiated with two to three daily high-protein nutritional drinks and iron, zinc, magnesia, B vitamins and vitamin D. She was referred for upper endoscopy for variceal status and for routine psychometric testing but did not show up.

Summer 2017

Six months after diagnosis it was noted by the outpatient nurse that she seemed beside herself. A physician acquainted with the patient's usual appearance suspected that the behavioural changes were caused by grade 1 HE. He found her fully awake, oriented in own data, time and place, without neurological deficits upon clinical examination including balance problems. She had a high-frequency tremor—but not asterixis. She was maintaining alcohol abstinence, eating all meals, and had one daily bowl movement. She was referred for psychometric testing to qualify and quantify cerebral deficits. A CT scan of the cerebrum was planned to rule out organic brain disease, i.e. stroke, haemorrhage and hygromas, as alternative explanations for her subtle behavioural change. At this point the patient continued to drive her car on a daily basis and was dependent on it to go shopping and for hospital visits. Her children did not show up for hospital visits.

The patient showed up a day late for the psychometric testing, driving her car and parking it in the middle of the parking lot entrapping several other cars. She told the outpatient nurse that it was impossible for her to attend testing the day before due to severe leg tremor. Also, she had not been mentally able to telephone to let us know that she was feeling beside herself.

Psychometric tests (PSE and CRT) were both abnormal (0.7 and −10), supporting the clinical impression of HE. The CT scan of the cerebrum eventually showed mild cerebral atrophy and signs of small prior cerebral insults. Standard biochemistry panel revealed slightly elevated CRP, a stable but slightly lowered sodium level, and venous ammonia level within normal range. It was concluded that the patient had grade 1 hepatic encephalopathy in addition to mild organic brain damage—the latter a stable condition most likely caused by her year-long alcohol overuse and small ischemic cerebral insults. Her HE was the most likely cause for the day-to-day fluctuations in cognitive capacity and we proceeded by seeking out modifiable precipitating factors.

Because of the elevated CRP ongoing bacterial infections were ruled out by blood and urine culturing, diagnostic paracentesis and a thorough dental examination. No infectious focus was found. Further, a recent abdominal CT scan was re-evaluated for large, treatable, porto-venous shunting. None were found. The patient was put on lactulose treatment, initially 10 mL bid. The outpatient nurse carefully communicated to municipal home caregivers that the patient had HE and lactulose was administered to ameliorate this, and not primarily as a laxative, and that the treatment goal was two to three bowl movements per day. Also, the nurse recommended the patient be given help to administer medicine and to have a daily visit to follow up on her brain function. The patient and her son were informed that she was unfit to drive her car for the time being.

Autumn 2017

During the following weeks the lactulose dose was titrated by the home-care nurse to 10 mL three times per day resulting in four bowl movements per day. The psychometric tests were repeated after 6 weeks and significant improvement was seen in the CRT index (1.2) but not in the PHES (−15). She remained oriented to date, time and place and abstinent from alcohol. Sodium levels remained normal and stable. The tremor was still present. It was decided to add rifaximin 550 mg bid and conduct new psychometric testing after 2 months.

Winter 2017

The patient returned for psychometric testing. She looked well nourished, was composed and could account for her future appointments with us. The psychometric tests had further improved: CRT index 1.5 and PHES −5. We decided to keep the patient on lactulose and rifaximin and retest within a few months hoping that she would improve further although given her underlying organic brain disease there might not be potential for further improvement.

Case 2: Recurrent HE with Co-morbid Medical Diseases

The patient, a 77-year male, was diagnosed with cryptogenic liver cirrhosis in 2006 after an upper GI bleed, which turned out to be caused by variceal bleeding. He completed a banding programme and was put on propranolol prophylaxis. Abdominal ultrasound revealed a cirrhotic liver and ascites for which he was treated with diuretics. The patient underwent routine psychometric testing using CRT test and was found to have stable reaction times and a high CRT index of 3.0 (Fig. 4.2, panel a).

The patient was highly educated, used to juggling several tasks at a time and handling a variety of electronic devices. He lived with his wife in a large villa, and had no need for help in daily activities and a full social life. We considered him as having a good cognitive reserve.

In spite of propranolol prophylaxis a new variceal bleed occurred in 2011 as a consequence of a portal vein thrombosis. Consequently the patient experienced a clinically manifest episode of hepatic encephalopathy requiring rehospitalisation. Lactulose treatment was initiated but unfortunately a new HE episode caused by lactulose-induced diarrhoea and dehydration occurred only 1 month later. Lactulose treatment was stopped at this point.

During the following 5 years the patient was diagnosed with type II diabetes, chronic obstructive lung disease and congestive heart failure. Further, he suffered recurring urinary tract infections. He had numerous hospital admissions each year. The patient was followed up regularly in the outpatient liver clinic: liver function remained stable (Child-Pugh class B) and ascites was controlled with varying doses of diuretics. Sodium levels were always within normal range but a slow decline in creatinine clearance was observed—we suspected it was owed to the increasing doses of diuretics necessary to rid the patient of recurring cardiogenic oedemas. Urine sodium was normal and hepato-renal syndrome was not suspected. The patient was always eloquent and seemed composed at clinical encounters albeit marked by his chronic conditions, and was always accompanied by his wife.

Upon enquiry, his wife shared with us that she found it difficult to keep track of all the ongoing appointments and treatments. The patient himself certainly could not manage this anymore—but what troubled her the most was the rapid fluctuation in the patient's mood and cognitive capacity. She felt very unsafe by this. One day the patient would be able to participate in daily activities while on the following day will be incontinent, tearful, sleep disturbed, and unable to use his mobile phone, turn on the TV or even move around without his walker. It had been going on and getting worse for several months. His wife told us about their home situation only when asked and although we knew the patient quite well we, as professionals, were not able to detect these problems.

Based on the wife's description of the patient we suspected he had HE, fluctuating between MHE and grade 2. The patient then went through neurological and psychometric evaluation. No neurological deficits were found at gross examination but the psychometric testing revealed a CRT index of 0.97 (Fig. 4.2, panel b), i.e. seriously unstable reaction times. The PHES was −7 and clearly abnormal. MMSE was normal indicating that the patient remained oriented and had no major memory problems, i.e. dementia. Venous ammonia levels were high within normal range on several occasions. A CT scan of the cerebrum and abdomen was performed and ruled out organic brain disease and large port-venous shunts. CRP was slightly elevated. Blood and urine culturing, diagnostic paracentesis and a dentist check were done to detect any asymptomatic bacterial infection. The urine turned out positive for *Enterococcus faecalis*. We concluded that the patient was clearly encephalopathic as judged by the abnormal psychometric testing; and that liver disease could in part explain this finding. At the same time, however, it was obvious that chronic infection, heart failure, progressive renal failure and diabetes also contributed to the overall decline in cerebral functioning. The hepatic component of his encephalopathy was perhaps even of lesser importance in the bigger picture. Of all the co-morbidities only the infection was modifiable and we initiated continuous treatment with antibiotics. After 1 month there was no longer bacteriuria. Significant improvement in CRT index (1.2) was found while the PHES improved to −5. His wife reported that sleep disturbances and incontinence episodes had improved.

He was scheduled for new testing after another month where the CRT index was found stable at 1.1 and PHES stable at −5. We decided to initiate anti-HE treatment seeking to further improve the patient's cerebral functions well aware that we would only see improvement if HE was a significant factor. The patient was known to be very sensitive to lactulose therapy (cf. above) so he was started on a low dose of lactulose of 10 mL bid and in addition a reduced dose of 550 mg of rifaximin (poor kidney function) to maximise the chance of effect in spite of relative lactulose intolerance.

He was scheduled for new testing after 2 months. At this occasion CRT index had improved further to the lowest normal value of 1.9 and PHES gone up to −4. The patient himself informed us that he had started using his cell phone again and his wife seconded that the patient was participating more in daily doings. We concluded that there was clearly an effect of the ammonia-lowering treatment and this was therefore continued.

Shortly thereafter an episode of clinically manifest HE grade 3 precipitated by dehydration after an increase in diuretics set the patient seriously back. Although he mentally cleared up within a few days he was readmitted shortly thereafter because his wife found him in a disoriented state. Upon admittance, however, he did not seem overtly encephalopathic. In the recognition that the patient's fragile and rapidly fluctuating cerebral functioning made it impossible for his wife to care for him at home he accepted moving into a nursing home where 24-h care was available. He continued lactulose and rifaximin.

The Impact of Minimal and Grade 1 HE

Overall, HE is the most debilitating manifestation of liver cirrhosis [17] and even in its mildest forms it heavily impacts patients' and caregivers' lives. MHE is present in approximately half of cirrhosis patients at any given point; and MHE patients are at higher risk of future clinically manifest HE as half will progress to develop overt HE requiring hospitalisation [6, 18, 19].

MHE also impacts the lives of patients in less visible ways: Slow psychomotor speed, attention deficits and problems in executive functions caused by MHE lead to a loss of practical and mental skills with detrimental consequences for patients and caregiver that can go unnoticed by professionals unless actively sought for. As illustrated by Case 2 we cannot count on the patient and caregiver to inform us of altered home functioning. This reluctance to share personal information is most likely owed to a fear of stigmatisation or simply lacking insight as to the connection between liver disease and brain dysfunction [20].

One of the well-documented, but less visible, effects of MHE is the negative impact on quality of life (QoL) in patients and caregivers [21–23]. The poor quality of life arises because the loss of skills caused by MHE results in a sense of altered identity, social isolation, dependence on others, sadness and anxiety [20, 24]. In Case 1 the patient's lacking ability to pick up the phone and call to inform us that she was feeling unwell illustrates the rapid onset of loss of skill. In Case 2 it is illustrated how HE impinges on the caregiver, as she has to take over the planning of hospital visits, help during incontinence episodes and live with the constant fear of the next HE bout, the latter ultimately resulting in the patient moving to a 24-h facility.

Fitness to drive is another skill often impacted by MHE, e.g. Case 1. Although not all MHE patients are unfit drivers, studies suggest that up to 50% may be judged both by performance during driving simulation and real-world traffic violations [3, 25–27]. This underlines the importance of obtaining driving history and of being familiar with the legal aspects involved in ensuing a driving ban. The topic is sensitive to many patients and physicians and often avoided because a driving ban severely limits patient autonomy [13].

MHE also leads to balance problems and a resulting increased risk of falls [4, 28, 29]. In a well-conducted Spanish study, the 1-year probability of falling was >50% for patients with liver cirrhosis and brain dysfunction as judged by the PHES vs. 6.5% in cirrhotic patients with normal PHES results [29]. Hence, taking measures to prevent falls could be worth considering, e.g. equipping the patient with a walker (Case 2), removing loose carpets and minimising the use of psychoactive drugs [30].

Diagnosing Minimal and Grade 1 Hepatic Encephalopathy

MHE poses a heavy burden; it is prevalent but treatable and consequently it is recommended to refer all patients with liver cirrhosis for psychometric testing at the time of diagnosis [1, 2, 23].

In the routine screening for MHE it is important to realise that the point at which MHE becomes detectable differs between patients depending on the daily requirements for brain functioning and the patients' cognitive reserve. In Case 1 the daily requirements for brain functioning are low: The patient has no job and no close relatives to hold her accountable for completing house chores. Hence MHE goes undetected until the point of her not being able to make a telephone call or park her car. In Case 2 the patient's environment, i.e. his fully active wife and his habitus for using rather advanced technology, requires a high level of brain functioning and thus MHE is detected at an earlier stage by caregivers. Conversely, upon psychometric testing, the patient with good cognitive reserve (Case 2) might be able to compensate for MHE masking and delaying the effects of MHE, while the patient with a poor cognitive reserve (Case 1) will have fewer compensatory mechanisms and is diagnosable with psychometry at the slightest brain impairment [15, 16].

Despite these differences in cognitive reserve both cases illustrate how psychometric tests help measure, i.e. standardise and objectify, defined brain functions; to relate them to healthy populations; and to monitor occurrence and development of the measured brain function. The tests are able, each in its own way, to detect the slowing of psychomotor speed, and the deficits in attention and executive functions, associated with HE. Preferably, two test modalities should be applied in order to measure as many aspects of brain functioning as possible since MHE affects different cognitive domains in different patients [1]. In an optimal situation the PSE test is used in combination with another locally validated test, i.e. spectral EEG (cf. Chap. 8), continuous reaction time test, critical flicker frequency measurement, inhibitory control test or the Stroop test [31–33].

None of these sensitive psychometric or neuropsychiatric tests are however specific to MHE; and good sensitivity and low specificity pose a risk of false-positive results. In the context of MHE specificity and positive predictive value are improved by applying the tests in high-risk populations, i.e. in patients with unequivocal signs of liver cirrhosis, and by creating an overview of competing causes for brain dysfunction.

Information obtained from the patient and caregivers will provide the necessary overview of these competing causes crucial to our interpretation of psychometric test results. Firstly, we make sure that the patient is oriented in time and place—if not, then brain dysfunction is equivalent to at least HE grade 2. Secondly, to form an idea of the patient's cognitive reserve or cognitive prerequisite, we enquire about educational level; current employment status; driving history; self-sufficiency/daily functioning level; use of psychoactive medications; substance abuse; prior cerebral events, i.e. strokes and seizures; and co-morbid diseases, i.e. heart failure, diabetes and chronic obstructive pulmonary disease which are competing causers of metabolic encephalopathy [7]. Whenever possible caregivers should accompany the patient to the clinic to back up or adjust the patient's story. Neurological examination should also be preformed.

The importance of maintaining an overview of competing causes is illustrated in Case 2 where co-morbid medical diseases render cerebral function very fragile even in a patient with a good cognitive reserve. In his case we chose to optimise treatment of modifiable competing causes (bacteriuria) before ensuing ammonia-lowering treatment. But ultimately attempting ammonia-lowering treatment could be the only way of determining to which extent MHE is a co-culprit, i.e. achieve diagnostic specificity.

References

1. Vilstrup H, Amodio P, Bajaj J, Cordoba J, Ferenci P, Mullen KD, et al. Hepatic encephalopathy in chronic liver disease: 2014 Practice Guideline by the American Association for the Study of Liver Diseases and the European Association for the Study of the Liver. Hepatology. 2014;60(2):715–35.
2. Gluud LL, Vilstrup H, Morgan MY. The effect of treatment for hepatic encephalopathy with nonabsorbable disaccarides on morbidity and mortality in patients with cirrhosis: systematic review and meta-analysis. In: Jalan R, editor. EASL International Liver Congress 2015; Vienna. ILC 2015 Abstract Book: EASL; 2015. p. 175.
3. Lauridsen MM, Thacker LR, White MB, Unser A, Sterling RK, Stravitz RT, et al. In patients with cirrhosis, driving simulator performance is associated with real-life driving. Clin Gastroenterol Hepatol. 2016;14(5):747–52.
4. Yildirim M. Falls in patients with liver cirrhosis. Gastroenterol Nurs. 2017;40(4):306–10.
5. Lauridsen MM, Mikkelsen S, Svensson T, Holm J, Kluver C, Gram J, et al. The continuous reaction time test for minimal hepatic encephalopathy validated by a randomized controlled multi-modal intervention—a pilot study. PLoS One. 2017;12(10):e0185412.
6. Lauridsen MM, Schaffalitzky de Muckadell OB, Vilstrup H. Minimal hepatic encephalopathy characterized by parallel use of the continuous reaction time and portosystemic encephalopathy tests. Metab Brain Dis. 2015;30(5):1187–92.
7. Lauridsen MM, Poulsen L, Rasmussen CK, Hogild M, Nielsen MK, de Muckadell OB, et al. Effects of common chronic medical conditions on psychometric tests used to diagnose minimal hepatic encephalopathy. Metab Brain Dis. 2015;31(2):267–72.
8. Lauridsen MM, Frojk J, de Muckadell OB, Vilstrup H. Opposite effects of sleep deprivation on the continuous reaction times in patients with liver cirrhosis and normal persons. Metab Brain Dis. 2014;29(3):655–60.
9. Lauridsen MM, Thiele M, Kimer N, Vilstrup H. The continuous reaction times method for diagnosing, grading, and monitoring minimal/covert hepatic encephalopathy. Metab Brain Dis. 2013;28:231–4.

10. Lauridsen MM, Gronbaek H, Naeser EB, Leth ST, Vilstrup H. Gender and age effects on the continuous reaction times method in volunteers and patients with cirrhosis. Metab Brain Dis. 2012:27:559–65.
11. Lauridsen MM, Jepsen P, Vilstrup H. Critical flicker frequency and continuous reaction times for the diagnosis of minimal hepatic encephalopathy: a comparative study of 154 patients with liver disease. Metab Brain Dis. 2011;26(2):135–9.
12. Weissenborn K. Neuropsychological characterization of hepatic encephalopathy. J Hepatol. 2001;34:768–73.
13. Lauridsen MM, Bajaj JS. Hepatic encephalopathy treatment and driving: a continental divide. J Hepatol. 2015;63:287–8.
14. Schomerus H, Hamster W. Neuropsychological aspects of portal-systemic encephalopathy. Metab Brain Dis. 1998;13(4):361–77.
15. Amodio P, Montagnese S, Spinelli G, Schiff S, Mapelli D. Cognitive reserve is a resilience factor for cognitive dysfunction in hepatic encephalopathy. Metab Brain Dis. 2017;32(4):1287–93.
16. Patel AV, Wade JB, Thacker LR, Sterling RK, Siddiqui MS, Stravitz RT, et al. Cognitive reserve is a determinant of health-related quality of life in patients with cirrhosis, independent of covert hepatic encephalopathy and model for end-stage liver disease score. Clin Gastroenterol Hepatol. 2015;13(5):987–91.
17. Bajaj JS, Wade JB, Gibson DP, Heuman DM, Thacker LR, Sterling RK, et al. The multi-dimensional burden of cirrhosis and hepatic encephalopathy on patients and caregivers. Am J Gastroenterol. 2011;106(9):1646–53.
18. Jepsen P, Ott P, Andersen PK, Sorensen HT, Vilstrup H. Clinical course of alcoholic liver cirrhosis: a Danish population-based cohort study. Hepatology. 2010;51(5):1675–82.
19. Sharma P, Sharma BC, Agrawal A, Sarin SK. Primary prophylaxis of overt hepatic encephalopathy in patients with cirrhosis: an open labeled randomized controlled trial of lactulose versus no lactulose. J Gastroenterol Hepatol. 2012;27:1329–35.
20. Ladegaard Gronkjaer L, Hoppe Sehstedt T, Norlyk A, Vilstrup H. Overt hepatic encephalopathy experienced by individuals with cirrhosis: a qualitative interview study. Gastroenterol Nurs. 2017; https:// doi: 10.1097/SGA.0000000000000286. [Epub ahead of print]
21. Groeneweg M, Quero JC, De Bruijn I, Hartmann IJ, Essink-bot ML, Hop WC, et al. Subclinical hepatic encephalopathy impairs daily functioning. Hepatology. 1998;28(1):45–9.

22. Orr JG, Homer T, Ternent L, Newton J, McNeil CJ, Hudson M, et al. Health related quality of life in people with advanced chronic liver disease. J Hepatol. 2014;61(5):1158–65.

23. Marchesini G, Bianchi G, Amodio P, Salerno F, Merli M, Panella C, et al. Factors associated with poor health-related quality of life of patients with cirrhosis. Gastroenterology. 2001;120(1):170–8.

24. Barboza KC, Salinas LM, Sahebjam F, Jesudian AB, Weisberg IL, Sigal SH. Impact of depressive symptoms and hepatic encephalopathy on health-related quality of life in cirrhotic hepatitis C patients. Metab Brain Dis. 2016;31(4):869–80.

25. Kircheis G, Knoche A, Hilger N, Manhart F, Schnitzler A, Schulze H, et al. Hepatic encephalopathy and fitness to drive. Gastroenterology. 2009;137(5):1706–15.e1–9.

26. Wein C, Koch H, Popp B, Oehler G, Schauder P. Minimal hepatic encephalopathy impairs fitness to drive. Hepatology. 2004;39(3):739–45.

27. Bajaj JS, Saeian K, Schubert CM, Hafeezullah M, Franco J, Varma RR, et al. Minimal hepatic encephalopathy is associated with motor vehicle crashes: the reality beyond the driving test. Hepatology. 2009;50(4):1175–83.

28. Urios A, Mangas-Losada A, Gimenez-Garzo C, Gonzalez-Lopez O, Giner-Duran R, Serra MA, et al. Altered postural control and stability in cirrhotic patients with minimal hepatic encephalopathy correlate with cognitive deficits. Liver Int. 2017;37(7):1013–22.

29. Soriano G, Roman E, Cordoba J, Torrens M, Poca M, Torras X, et al. Cognitive dysfunction in cirrhosis is associated with falls: a prospective study. Hepatology. 2012;55(6):1922–30.

30. Tips for preventing falls. Am Fam Physician. 2017;96(4): https://www.aafp.org/afp/2017/0815/p240-s1.html

31. Bajaj JS, Heuman DM, Sterling RK, Sanyal AJ, Siddiqui M, Matherly S, et al. Validation of EncephalApp, Smartphone-Based Stroop Test, for the Diagnosis of Covert Hepatic Encephalopathy. Clin Gastroenterol Hepatol. 2015;13(10):1828–1835.e1.

32. Bajaj JS, Thacker LR, Heuman DM, Fuchs M, Sterling RK, Sanyal AJ, et al. The Stroop smartphone application is a short and valid method to screen for minimal hepatic encephalopathy. Hepatology. 2013;58(3):1122–32.

33. Kircheis G, Hilger N, Haussinger D. Value of critical flicker frequency and psychometric hepatic encephalopathy score in diagnosis of low-grade hepatic encephalopathy. Gastroenterology. 2014;146(4):961–9.

Chapter 5

Treatment Options for Covert Hepatic Encephalopathy

Sahaj Rathi and Radha K. Dhiman

Abbreviations

AASLD	American Association for the Study of Liver Diseases
BCAA	Branched-chain amino acids
CFF	Critical flicker frequency
CHE	Covert hepatic encephalopathy
EASL	European Association for the Study of the Liver
HE	Hepatic encephalopathy
LOLA	L-Ornithine L-aspartate
MELD	Model for end-stage liver disease
MMSE	Mini-mental state examination
OHE	Overt hepatic encephalopathy
PHES	Psychometric hepatic encephalopathy score
PSS	Portosystemic shunt
SBP	Spontaneous bacterial peritonitis

S. Rathi, M.D., D.M. · R. K. Dhiman, M.D.,D.M.,F.A.C.G.,F.A.A.S.L.D. (✉)
Department of Hepatology, Post Graduate Institute of Medical Education and Research, Chandigarh, India

© Springer International Publishing AG, part of Springer Nature 2018   65
J. S. Bajaj (ed.), *Diagnosis and Management of Hepatic Encephalopathy*, https://doi.org/10.1007/978-3-319-76798-7_5

Clinical Vignette

Case 1

A 45-year-old male with a history of ethanol-related cirrhosis for the past 3 years presented for routine follow-up. He was doing well on medical management and had no episodes of overt encephalopathy, ascites, jaundice, or variceal bleeding. His only complaint was a feeling of fatigue. Upon questioning he admitted being "a little careless" lately. He had been in a minor traffic accident last month due to inattention. Family members reported him to be a "very careful" driver in the past. Clinical examination was unremarkable except a palpable spleen. His mini-mental state examination (MMSE) was normal, and he could perform simple calculations. His Child-Pugh score was 6/15 (Child class A), and MELD score was 8. A psychometric hepatic encephalopathy score (PHES) battery and critical flicker frequency(CFF) test were done under a study protocol, which revealed evidence of covert hepatic encephalopathy (CHE) (PHES −8; CFF 34/s).

Case 2

A 64-year-old lady with cryptogenic cirrhosis for the past 2 years, which has been well compensated, was admitted for Colles' fracture. She had history of another fall a couple of weeks back which led to a knee bruise. There was no history of behavioral changes or disorientation. A detailed neurological examination including MMSE was unremarkable. Her Sickness Impact Profile-Covert Hepatic Encephalopathy (SIP-CHE) score was 2, indicating covert HE. She also performed poorly on the animal naming test (10 in 1 min). Covert HE was confirmed by administering PHES battery.

Hepatic encephalopathy (HE) is one of the most troublesome complications of cirrhosis. It affects a majority of patients at some point during the course of disease. The spectrum of neurological involvement is diverse, ranging from subtle cognitive changes to deep coma. Based upon the severity of neurological deficit, HE has been subdivided into overt and covert. Overt HE is when the encephalopathy is evident on a physician evaluation. Patients with more subtle cognitive changes inapparent on a routine clinical examination are categorized as covert HE—a term which includes both minimal HE and Grade I HE of the West Haven scale.

Covert HE (CHE) may be seen in 30–84% patients with cirrhosis [1]. Cognitive defects in these patients include inattention, impaired visuomotor coordination, and impaired working memory. These changes result in poor quality of life, driving difficulties, accident proneness, and workspace problems [1]. Patients with CHE are more likely to develop progression of cirrhosis, episodes of overt HE, and mortality [2, 3]. The implications are not limited to the patient, as CHE is also associated with an increased burden on the caregivers [4]. However, this condition is highly under-recognized and undertreated due to the paucity of evident symptoms and absence of standard definitions. The diagnosis of covert HE is based upon specialized neurocognitive testing, and is covered in another chapter in this book.

Treatment of CHE predominantly revolves around lowering ammonia levels, even though neuroinflammation and oxidative stress too contribute to CHE. Agents that reduce ammonia include nonabsorbable disaccharides, antibiotics, ammonia scavengers, nutritional modulation, and probiotics. However, unlike overt HE, trials in covert HE are relatively limited.

Nonabsorbable Disaccharides

Nonabsorbable disaccharides like lactulose and lactitol have been the mainstay of therapy in patients with hepatic encephalopathy for decades. They lead to reversal of CHE as evidenced by improvement in psychometric scores, thereby improving health-related quality of life. They also prevent development of overt episodes of hepatic encephalopathy [5–7]. In a placebo-controlled trial, treatment with lactulose for 3 months led to reduction in the number of abnormal neurophysiological tests and improvement in quality of life [6]. The use of lactulose has been considered cost effective in preventing motor vehicle accidents in the United States [8]. However, the existing evidence does not yet support improvement in driving performance with lactulose.

The major side effects of this drug include diarrhea, bloating, and nausea. Most studies from the Eastern parts of the world report very low rates of drug discontinuation due to side effects, while these numbers may be up to 28% in the West [9, 10]. These side effects are usually dose dependent, and can be minimized by titrating doses to achieve two three soft stools per day. We have recently shown that sociocultural factors play a major role in patient acceptance of lactulose and perception of its side effects. We projected risk-benefit scenarios of chances of developing OHE against expected side effects of lactulose to two cohorts of patients, one each from India and the United States. Indian patients were much more likely to accept lactulose even if the risk of OHE was low, probably as twice-a-day stool frequency is considered acceptable in India [11].

Antibiotics

Rifaximin has replaced metronidazole and neomycin as the antibiotic of choice in the management of HE. It is a nonabsorbable antibiotic which modulates gut flora and improves dysbiosis. Moreover, rifaximin has not been shown to induce resistance in the intestinal flora, and has very rarely been associated with *Clostridium difficile*-associated diarrhea [12].

Rifaximin has been effective in the improvement of psychometric scores, thereby reversing CHE. It also improves quality of life and driving performance in patients with CHE. It is usually well tolerated, and drug discontinuation is rarely required [13, 14].

Probiotics

The ratio of autochthonous to non-autochthonous flora significantly affect ammoniagenesis. Probiotics have been shown to improve HE by reducing gut dysbiosis. Both pharmaceutical probiotic preparations and commercially available probiotic yogurt have been studied in this regard [15, 16]. These have been successful in reversing CHE and improving quality of life while being well tolerated by most. A recent meta-analysis suggested that probiotics led to improvement in CHE and reduced recurrence of OHE [17].

Ammonia Scavengers

L-Ornithine-L-aspartate stimulates urea cycle and glutamine synthesis in the periportal hepatocytes and skeletal muscles, consuming ammonia in the process. It has been effective in reversal of CHE, improving quality of life, as well as prevention of OHE [7, 18].

Nutrition

Cirrhosis is a state of accelerated starvation as a consequence of depleted hepatic glycogen stores, deficient muscle stores due to sarcopenia, and systemic inflammation. As a result, a majority of patients exhibit features of malnutrition [19]. Protein restriction in patients with encephalopathy is not recommended anymore. Cirrhotic patients seem to have better cognitive function in a fed state as opposed to a fasting state despite higher ammonia levels in the latter [20]. A recent trial demonstrated that patients compliant with a diet of 30–35 kcal/kg/day energy and 1.0–1.5 g/kg/day vegetable protein intake showed reversal of CHE and improvement in quality of life. This effect was more pronounced in patients with early cirrhosis [21]. The use of branched-chain amino acids as dietary supplements has also been associated with CHE reversal and increased muscle mass [22].

Shunt Closure

Presence of spontaneous portosystemic shunts may predispose cirrhotic as well as noncirrhotic patients for CHE. This has been demonstrated in patients with extrahepatic portal venous obstruction and noncirrhotic portal fibrosis where evidence of cognitive deficit is present despite normal hepatocellular synthetic function [23, 24]. However, currently there is neither evidence nor recommendation to suggest occlusion of these shunts in such situations for CHE.

Fecal Microbiota Transplantation (FMT)

Gut microbiota modulation with antibiotics and pre/probiotics has long been used for treatment of HE. An attempt to modulate gut microbiome with FMT made in a patient with CHE who was unable to afford standard therapy showed improvement in cognition with FMT [25]. Thereafter, a randomized controlled trial showed lower rates of HE recurrence and improved cognition in patients who received FMT, while there was no change in the overall MELD score. Moreover, the FMT group had lower frequency of severe adverse events. However, larger, well-controlled trials are needed to establish safety and efficacy before FMT can be recommended as a treatment option [26].

Approach Considerations

A paucity of studies in general, and well-controlled head-to-head trials in particular, limit informed decision-making when choosing the appropriate agent and duration of therapy in patients with CHE. Considering this, we recently conducted a network meta-analysis to compare the efficacies of all available agents. Such analysis can give meaningful comparisons between pharmaceutical agents which have not been compared head to head, with the help of appropriate statistical tools. In this study, rifaximin and lactulose were found to be the most effective agents for reversal of CHE [27].

Whether all patients with CHE need treatment is a matter of debate among the experts. Whereas many studies support treating CHE by demonstrating improvement in quality of life, cognitive function, and driving performance, the heterogeneity in the diagnostic criteria used, short follow-up, and lack of clinically relevant endpoints limit the significance of this evidence. The 2014 EASL-AASLD guidelines do not recommend treatment of CHE routinely due to a paucity of robust evidence of benefit. This conclusion was derived largely based on studies about MHE. Nevertheless, the negative implications of CHE on the quality of life, work performance, driving, and caregiver burden are well described. While patients categorized as grade I HE may be treated routinely, the decision of treating those with minimal HE is better taken on a case-to-case basis after a thorough discussion with the patient. The anticipated benefits have to be carefully weighed against the adverse effects of medications and cost of therapy. Patients who drive for a living, operate heavy machinery, have a history of accidents/falls which can be ascribed to inattention, or complain of reduced work productivity may be routinely treated.

No recommendations exist on the duration of treatment in these patients. Most studies have continued treatment for 3–6 months. However, follow-up data is not available for these patients. A recently published research followed up patients for 6 months after 3 months of lactulose or rifaximin therapy. They found that over half of the patients, who initially had resolution of CHE, had an episode of OHE or developed CHE again after discontinuation [28]. As the underlying disease persists, it may thus be prudent to continue the therapy indefinitely or until tolerated in order to maintain the non-encephalopathic state (Fig. 5.1).

Clinical Vignette: Follow-Up

Case 1

The patient was started on appropriate nutritional therapy with high-protein (vegetable and casein based) diet ~1 g/kg/day, and energy intake of ~35 kcal/kg/day. Rifaximin 550 mg twice daily was started as the patient was unwilling for lactulose therapy. The patient was reassessed 3 months later. He reported feeling more energetic. His psychometric scores and quality-of-life parameters improved. However, there was no change in the Child-Pugh or MELD scores. He has not had any further accidents since the beginning of therapy, and is tolerating the therapy well.

Case 2

The patient underwent surgical fixation of the fracture. After the surgery, her nutrition was optimized with a high-protein and high-calorie diet (as in Case 1). In addition, branched-chain amino acids were supplemented. On follow-up 3 months later, she had no further falls, reported subjective improvement in well-being, and showed an improvement in her PHES score.

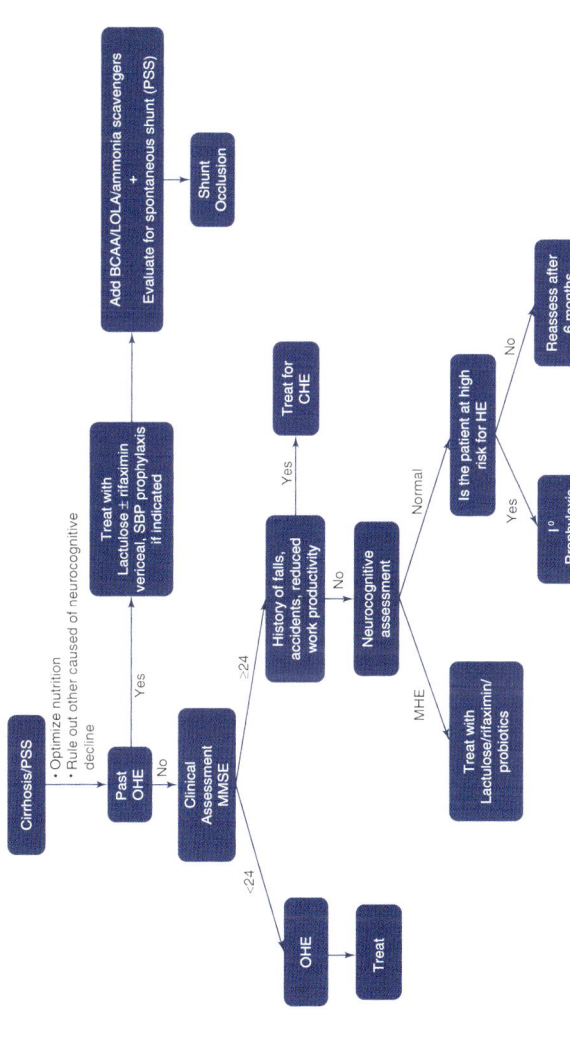

Fig. 5.1 Algorithm for outpatient management of hepatic encephalopathy. *BCAA* branched-chain amino acids. *LOLA* L-ornithine L-aspartate. *MMSE* mini-mental state examination. *PSS* portosystemic shunting. *SBP* spontaneous bacterial peritonitis. Source: From Ref. [29]

References

1. Dhiman RK, Chawla YK. Minimal hepatic encephalopathy. Indian J Gastroenterol. 2009;28(1):5–16. https://doi.org/10.1007/s12664-009-0003-6.
2. Dhiman RK, Kurmi R, Thumburu KK, et al. Diagnosis and prognostic significance of minimal hepatic encephalopathy in patients with cirrhosis of liver. Dig Dis Sci. 2010;55(8):2381–90. https://doi.org/10.1007/s10620-010-1249-7.
3. Ampuero J, Montoliú C, Simón-Talero M, et al. Minimal hepatic encephalopathy identifies patients at risk of faster cirrhosis progression. J Gastroenterol Hepatol. 2017. https://doi.org/10.1111/jgh.13917.
4. Bajaj JS, Wade JB, Gibson DP, et al. The multi-dimensional burden of cirrhosis and hepatic encephalopathy on patients and caregivers. Am J Gastroenterol. 2011;106(9):1646–53. https://doi.org/10.1038/ajg.2011.157.
5. Dhiman RK, Sawhney MS, Chawla YK, Das G, Ram S, Dilawari JB. Efficacy of lactulose in cirrhotic patients with subclinical hepatic encephalopathy. Dig Dis Sci. 2000;45(8):1549–52. http://www.ncbi.nlm.nih.gov/pubmed/11007104. Accessed 27 Oct 2017
6. Prasad S, Dhiman RK, Duseja A, Chawla YK, Sharma A, Agarwal R. Lactulose improves cognitive functions and health-related quality of life in patients with cirrhosis who have minimal hepatic encephalopathy. Hepatology. 2007;45(3):549–59. https://doi.org/10.1002/hep.21533.
7. Mittal VV, Sharma BC, Sharma P, Sarin SK. A randomized controlled trial comparing lactulose, probiotics, and L-ornithine L-aspartate in treatment of minimal hepatic encephalopathy. Eur J Gastroenterol Hepatol. 2011;23(8):725–32. https://doi.org/10.1097/MEG.0b013e32834696f5.
8. Bajaj JS, Pinkerton SD, Sanyal AJ, Heuman DM. Diagnosis and treatment of minimal hepatic encephalopathy to prevent motor vehicle accidents: a cost-effectiveness analysis. Hepatology. 2012;55(4):1164–71. https://doi.org/10.1002/hep.25507.
9. Bajaj JS, Sanyal AJ, Bell D, Gilles H, Heuman DM. Predictors of the recurrence of hepatic encephalopathy in lactulose-treated patients. Aliment Pharmacol Ther. 2010;31(9):1012–7. https://doi.org/10.1111/j.1365-2036.2010.04257.x.

10. Sharma BC, Sharma P, Agrawal A, Sarin SK. Secondary prophylaxis of hepatic encephalopathy: an open-label randomized controlled trial of lactulose versus placebo. Gastroenterology. 2009;137(3):885–91, 891.e1. https://doi.org/10.1053/j.gastro.2009.05.056.
11. Rathi S, Fagan A, Wade J, et al. Lactulose acceptance varies between Indian and American covert HE patients: implications for comparing, designing and interpreting global HE trials. J Clin Exp Hepatol. 2017;7:S51–2. https://doi.org/10.1016/j.jceh.2017.01.067.
12. Bajaj JS, Heuman DM, Sanyal AJ, et al. Modulation of the metabiome by rifaximin in patients with cirrhosis and minimal hepatic encephalopathy. PLoS One. 2013;8(4):e60042. https://doi.org/10.1371/journal.pone.0060042.
13. Sidhu SS, Goyal O, Mishra BP, Sood A, Chhina RS, Soni RK. Rifaximin improves psychometric performance and health-related quality of life in patients with minimal hepatic encephalopathy (the RIME trial). Am J Gastroenterol. 2011;106(2):307–16. https://doi.org/10.1038/ajg.2010.455.
14. Bajaj JS, Heuman DM, Wade JB, et al. Rifaximin improves driving simulator performance in a randomized trial of patients with minimal hepatic encephalopathy. Gastroenterology. 2011;140(2):478–487.e1. https://doi.org/10.1053/j.gastro.2010.08.061.
15. Dhiman RK, Rana B, Agrawal S, et al. Probiotic VSL#3 reduces liver disease severity and hospitalization in patients with cirrhosis: a randomized, controlled trial. Gastroenterology. 2014;147(6):1327–1337.e3. https://doi.org/10.1053/j.gastro.2014.08.031.
16. Bajaj JS, Saeian K, Christensen KM, et al. Probiotic yogurt for the treatment of minimal hepatic encephalopathy. Am J Gastroenterol. 2008;103(7):1707–15. https://doi.org/10.1111/j.1572-0241.2008.01861.x.
17. Dalal R, Mcgee RG, Riordan SM, Webster AC. Probiotics for people with hepatic encephalopathy. Cochrane Database Syst Rev. 2017;(2). https://doi.org/10.1002/14651858.CD008716.pub3.
18. Sharma K, Pant S, Misra S, et al. Effect of rifaximin, probiotics, and l-ornithine l-aspartate on minimal hepatic encephalopathy: a randomized controlled trial. Saudi J Gastroenterol. 2014;20(4):225. https://doi.org/10.4103/1319-3767.136975.
19. Chadalavada R, Biyyani RSS, Maxwell J, Mullen K. Nutrition in hepatic encephalopathy. Nutr Clin Pract. 2010;25(3):257–64. https://doi.org/10.1177/0884533610368712.

20. Vaisman N, Katzman H, Carmiel-Haggai M, Lusthaus M, Niv E. Breakfast improves cognitive function in cirrhotic patients with cognitive impairment. Am J Clin Nutr. 2010;92(1):137–40. https://doi.org/10.3945/ajcn.2010.29211.

21. Maharshi S, Sharma BC, Sachdeva S, Srivastava S, Sharma P. Efficacy of nutritional therapy for patients with cirrhosis and minimal hepatic encephalopathy in a randomized trial. Clin Gastroenterol Hepatol. 2016;14(3):454–460.e3.; quiz e33. https://doi.org/10.1016/j.cgh.2015.09.028.

22. Les I, Doval E, García-Martínez R, et al. Effects of branched-chain amino acids supplementation in patients with cirrhosis and a previous episode of hepatic encephalopathy: a randomized study. Am J Gastroenterol. 2011;106(6):1081–8. https://doi.org/10.1038/ajg.2011.9.

23. Sharma P, Sharma BC, Puri V, Sarin SK. Natural history of minimal hepatic encephalopathy in patients with extrahepatic portal vein obstruction. Am J Gastroenterol. 2009;104(4):885–90. https://doi.org/10.1038/ajg.2009.84.

24. Das K, Singh P, Chawla Y, Duseja A, Dhiman RK, Suri S. Magnetic resonance imaging of brain in patients with cirrhotic and non-cirrhotic portal hypertension. Dig Dis Sci. 2008;53(10):2793–8. https://doi.org/10.1007/s10620-008-0383-y.

25. Kao D, Roach B, Park H, et al. Fecal microbiota transplantation in the management of hepatic encephalopathy. Hepatology. 2016;63(1):339–40. https://doi.org/10.1002/hep.28121.

26. Bajaj JS, Kassam Z, Fagan A, et al. Fecal microbiota transplant from a rational stool donor improves hepatic encephalopathy: a randomized clinical trial. Hepatology. 2017. https://doi.org/10.1002/hep.29306.

27. Thumburu KK, Dhiman RK, Chopra M, et al. Comparative effectiveness of different pharmacological interventions for the treatment of minimal hepatic encephalopathy: a systematic review with network meta-analysis. J Clin Exp Hepatol. 2017;7:S6–7. https://doi.org/10.1016/j.jceh.2017.01.010.

28. Goyal O, Sidhu S, Kishore H. Minimal hepatic encephalopathy in cirrhosis—how long to treat? Ann Hepatol. 2017;16(1):115–22. https://doi.org/10.5604/16652681.1226822.

29. Rathi S, Dhiman RK. Managing encephalopathy in the outpatient setting. Clin Liver Dis. 2016;8(6):150–5. https://doi.org/10.1002/cld.590.

Chapter 6
Latest Concepts in Inpatient Hepatic Encephalopathy Management

Thoetchai (Bee) Peeraphatdit, Patrick S. Kamath, and Michael D. Leise

Abbreviations

ACLF	Acute-on-chronic liver failure
BCAA	Branched-chain amino acids
CLIF-C ACLF	Chronic Liver Failure Consortium ACLF Score
DAMPs	Damage-associated molecular patterns
ESPEN	European Society for Parenteral and Enteral Nutrition
FDA	Food and Drug Administration
HE	Hepatic encephalopathy
IL	Interleukin
LOLA	L-ornithine L-aspartate
LT	Liver transplant
MARS	Molecular adsorbent recirculating system

T. Peeraphatdit, M.D. · P. S. Kamath, M.D. (✉) · M. D. Leise, M.D.
Division of Gastroenterology and Hepatology, Mayo Clinic College of
Medicine, Rochester, MN, USA
e-mail: peeraphatdit.thoetchai@mayo.edu; Kamath.patrick@mayo.edu;
Leise.michael@mayo.edu

© Springer International Publishing AG, part of Springer Nature 2018   77
J. S. Bajaj (ed.), *Diagnosis and Management of Hepatic
Encephalopathy*, https://doi.org/10.1007/978-3-319-76798-7_6

MELD   Model for end-stage liver disease
PAMPs   Pathogen-associated molecular patterns
RCT   Randomized controlled trial
TIPS   Transjugular intrahepatic portosystemic
                  shunt

Patient Scenario 1

A 35-year-old female with past medical history of compensated alcoholic cirrhosis presented with altered mental status after alcohol binge drinking. On physical exam, her vital signs were stable. She was only oriented to self and had marked jaundice and asterixis. Her laboratory result showed leukocyte count of 15×10^9/L, creatinine of 5.7 mg/dL (with baseline of 1.0 mg/dL), aspartate aminotransferase of 288 U/L, alanine aminotransferase of 119 U/L, alkaline phosphatase of 383 U/L, total bilirubin of 28.6 mg/dL, direct bilirubin of 23.8 mg/dL, and international normalized ratio of 3.1. Urinalysis showed pyuria and urine culture showed *Escherichia coli* >100,000 cfu/mL. She was diagnosed with hepatic encephalopathy (HE), urinary tract infection, severe alcoholic hepatitis, and acute-on-chronic liver failure.

Discussion

This patient had hepatic encephalopathy in a setting of acute-on-chronic liver failure (ACLF) given that she had acute renal injury as an extrahepatic organ failure. Patients with HE in the context of ACLF had a heightened risk of mortality compared to isolated HE. Thus, early detection of extrahepatic organ failure was vital for risk stratification purposes and to determine the need for organ support. Intensive care unit admission should be considered as she was likely to require renal replacement therapy. In addition, she would require treatment for severe alcoholic hepatitis and urinary tract infection, the precipitating factors for hepatic encephalopathy.

Patient Scenario 2

A 66-year-old female with decompensated nonalcoholic steato-hepatitis cirrhosis and chronic kidney disease presented with worsening altered mental status for 2 days. She had been compliant with the maintenance lactulose regimen that had been started after one prior episode of precipitated HE. Her vital sign demonstrated slight tachycardia with heart are of 114/min with normal blood pressure of 145/77 mmHg. Her oxygen saturation is 95% on room air. She was awake but confused and not able to answer any questions. Asterixis was noted. The white blood cell count was 8.5×10^9/L and the creatinine was at her baseline of 1.7 mg/dL. The microscopic urinalysis showed >50 white blood cells/high power field and the urine culture was positive for *Escherichia coli*.

Discussion

Because the patient did not have any other evidence of extrahepatic organ failure other than hepatic encephalopathy, she was diagnosed with isolated hepatic encephalopathy. Because she had recurrent episode of hepatic encephalopathy while on lactulose, rifaximin was added. In addition, the urinary tract infection which was the precipitating factor was treated.

Patient Scenario 3

A 65-year-old male with decompensated nonalcoholic steato-
hepatitis cirrhosis, model for end-stage liver disease (MELD)
score of 13, was admitted with persistent hepatic encephalopathy. He had multiple previous admissions for episodic overt
hepatic encephalopathy and no precipitating factors were identified. His examination was consistent with West Haven Criteria
(WHC) Grade 3 HE. He did not respond to lactulose, rifaximin,
and zinc therapy. Computed tomography of the abdomen with
intravenous contrast demonstrated a large splenorenal shunt.

Discussion

The patient should be considered for splenorenal shunt embolization for persistent HE not responding to medical treatment
and relatively low MELD score (MELD <15). Previous studies
showed that approximately 45–70% of patients with refractory
HE had large portosystemic shunts discovered on evaluation
and that the embolization of the portosystemic shunt was a safe
and effective treatment. The patient received the embolization
of the splenorenal shunt and his hepatic encephalopathy significantly improved.

Introduction

Hepatic encephalopathy (HE) is a major neuropsychiatric
abnormality seen in patients with decompensated cirrhosis or
portosystemic shunting. The clinical presentation ranges from
subtle brain function changes that require neuropsychometric
testing for diagnosis to a hepatic coma state. The severity of HE
can be graded into covert HE (West Haven criteria grade 0–1)

and overt HE (West Haven criteria grade 2–4). Most patients with overt HE will require inpatient management and this will be the focus for this chapter.

Overt HE occurs in approximately 30–45% of patients with cirrhosis and 10–60% of patients with transjugular portosystemic shunt (TIPS) [1–3]. In the US Nationwide Inpatient Sample, the national estimate of annual incidence of overt HE admission is 110,000–115,000. The average length of inpatient stay was 8.5 days and the average total inpatient charges were $63,108 per case [4]. Moreover, overt HE is associated with increased risk of mortality in hospitalized patients with cirrhosis independently of the severity of cirrhosis (adjusting for the MELD score) [5] or extrahepatic organ failures [6].

Management of the hospitalized patient with overt HE focuses on correcting the underlying precipitating factors and providing pharmacologic treatment that reduces ammoniagenesis. Most patients will require maintenance medication to prevent recurrence of HE and to prevent hospital readmission. The prevention of HE will be discussed in Chap. 7.

Hepatic Encephalopathy in Acute-on-Chronic Liver Failure

For the past two decades, the concept of acute-on-chronic liver failure (ACLF) has been proposed on the basis that patients with chronic liver disease or cirrhosis who developed acute unexpected hepatic decompensation and extrahepatic organ failure have significant increased risk of short-term mortality [7]. Three different definitions have been proposed from three different regions of the world [8–10]. The most current definition by a working group on behalf of the Working Party of the World Gastroenterology Organization is as follows: "ACLF is a syndrome in patients with chronic liver disease with or without previously diagnosed cirrhosis which is characterized by acute hepatic decompensation resulting in liver failure (jaundice and prolongation of the international normalized ratio) and one or more extrahepatic organ failures that is associated with increased mortality within a period of 28 days and up to 3 months from onset" [11].

The prevalence of ACLF is difficult to assess given the difference in the ACLF definition. In the European multicenter study, the prevalence among hospitalized cirrhotic patients with acute decompensation was 31% [8]. A study from US Nationwide Inpatient Sample reported ACLF prevalence of 5% among hospitalizations for cirrhosis in 2011 [12]. With the increase in ACLF recognition, there is an emerging concept that differentiates hepatic encephalopathy that occurs in the setting of decompensated cirrhosis from that arising in the context of ACLF.

Isolated Hepatic Encephalopathy

Isolated hepatic encephalopathy occurs in a setting of decompensated cirrhosis without evidence of extrahepatic organ dysfunction. Isolated hepatic encephalopathy seems to occur in older cirrhotic patients who are inactive drinkers. It is not clearly associated with hepatic dysfunction but rather develops in the setting of chronic diuretic use. There is no significant inflammatory reaction. The prognosis is good even in those requiring intensive care unit admission and mechanical ventilation for airway protection [13, 14].

Hepatic Encephalopathy Associated with Acute-on-Chronic Liver Failure

HE associated with ACLF occurs in the setting of extrahepatic organ failures. It seems to occur in young cirrhotic patients who

are active drinkers [14]. This type of HE is associated with
hepatic dysfunction and bacterial infections. In contrast with
isolated hepatic encephalopathy, HE associated with ACLF has
a grave prognosis. In addition to hyperammonemia that is
observed in both types of HE, the significant inflammatory
reaction found in ACLF may explain this prognostic gap [15].

Pathophysiology of Hepatic Encephalopathy in Acute-on-Chronic Liver Failure

Pathophysiology for HE is discussed in detail in Chaps. 2 and
3. In this chapter, we focus on the pathophysiology of HE in the
setting of ACLF. Jalan et al. proposed the pathophysiology of
ACLF using a four-part model of predisposing event, injury
resulting from precipitating event, response to injury, and organ
failure (Fig. 6.1) [7, 16]. Predisposition is the underlying

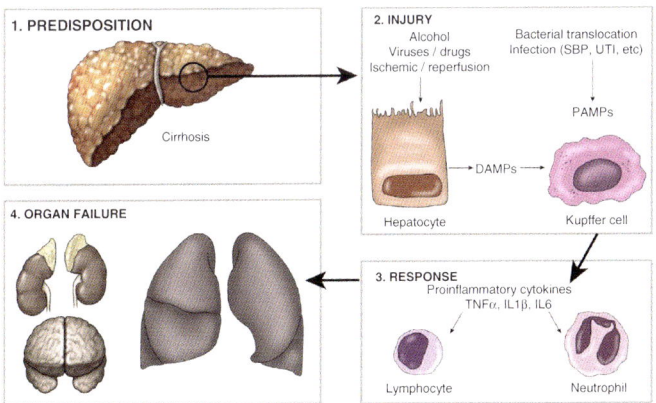

Fig. 6.1 Pathophysiology of ACLF. Asrani et al. 7. *PAMP* pathogen-associated molecular pattern, *SBP* spontaneous bacterial peritonitis, *TNF* tumor
necrosis factor, *UTI* urinary tract infection

chronic liver disease. Injury can be from multiple etiologies, e.g., bacterial infection, alcohol intake, viral hepatitis, reactivation of hepatitis B, gastrointestinal bleeding, drug-induced liver injury, ischemia, infection, or surgery. The inflammatory response is important as suggested by the presence of increased C-reactive protein and an increase in leukocyte count. In the setting of bacterial translocation, lipopolysaccharide and other pathogen-associated molecular patterns (PAMPs) trigger Kupffer cells to release proinflammatory cytokines, namely IL-1, IL-6, and tumor necrosis factor alpha, which induce inflammatory reaction by leukocyte recruitment and oxidative stress. In addition to bacterial translocation, sterile processes such as alcohol, ischemia, or surgery can elicit an inflammatory response by damaging hepatocytes and with subsequent release of damage-associated molecular patterns (DAMPs), Fig. 6.1 [17, 18]. Organ failure is the final step of the pathway. An increase in the number of organ failure is associated with increase in the mortality rate [8].

The pathophysiology of HE in ACLF is multifactorial and hyperammonemia and systemic inflammation are important factors [2]. Studies in animal models have shown that induction of hyperammonemia leads to brain edema and the reduction of ammonia level could reduce brain swelling [19]. In addition, reduction in ammonia level prevented brain edema and delayed the development of coma in response to LPS challenge in an animal model [20]. Clinically, HE associated with ACLF may lead to cerebral edema and increased intracranial pressure whereas isolated hepatic encephalopathy typically will not [21]. Cerebral edema has been observed in imaging studies [22] and confirmed by electron microscopic studies in animal models showing astrocyte swelling and collapsed microvessels [23].

Management of Hepatic Encephalopathy in the Hospitalized Patient

General Approach

Early risk stratification to differentiate isolated HE from HE associated with ACLF is necessary (Fig. 6.2). This is due to the significant difference in short-term mortality between these two groups [14]. Prognostic scores including the chronic liver failure-sequential organ failure assessment (CLIF-SOFA) score may be utilized to determine the severity of ACLF [8]. If HE

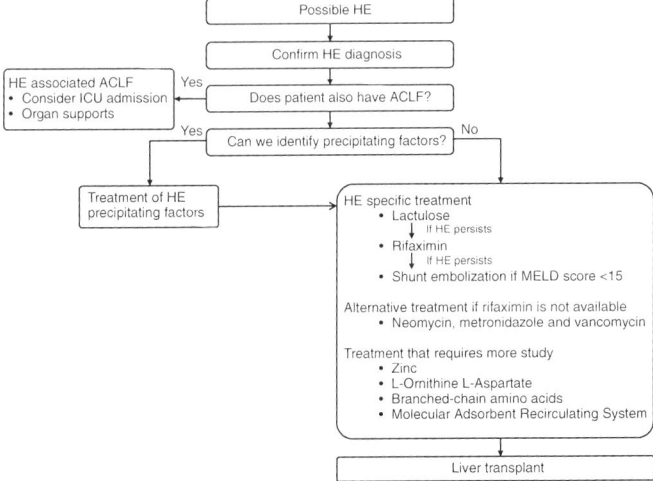

Fig. 6.2 Management of hospitalized patients with hepatic encephalopathy

associated with ACLF is detected, intensive care unit admission should be considered. Airway protection should be considered in all patients with grades 3–4 HE, particularly those with ACLF, or if there is evolving respiratory failure. Inotropes or vasopressors should be considered to maintain adequate cerebral perfusion.

In addition to the treatment of HE that is present at hospital admission, there is also a potential benefit from preventing the progression of HE. In a study from 1,560 patients from the North American Consortium for Study of End-stage Liver Disease evaluating hospitalized patients with cirrhosis, the maximum HE grade and not the admission HE grade was found to be prognostic for mortality independently of the extrahepatic organ failures [6].

Direct Treatment at Precipitating Factors

The most common precipitating factors of HE are diuretic use, bacterial infection, and alcohol use [14]. Any identifiable precipitating event should be promptly treated and early antibiotics administration should be considered when infection is suspected.

Specific Treatment

Nonabsorbable Disaccharides

Nonabsorbed disaccharides (e.g., lactulose and lactitol) and nonabsorbable antibiotics (e.g., neomycin and rifaximin) represent the mainstay of specific treatment for HE. Lactulose (b-galactosidofructose) and lactitol (b-galactosidosorbitol) reduce ammonia absorption in the colon by acidification of the colon resulting in the conversion of ammonia to ammonium, shifting the colonic flora from urease- to nonurease-producing bacterial species, and by their cathartic effect. A large meta-analysis in 2004 showed that nonabsorbable disaccharides were superior to placebo. However, when only high-quality trials were included, nonabsorbable disaccharides were found to have no effect on HE [24]. The inconsistent finding in this study is most likely explained by the heterogeneity of HE in previous nonabsorbable disaccharide clinical trials. For example, an overt HE episode may occur in the setting of acute liver failure, acute-on-chronic liver failure, or may be precipitated by a reversible precipitating factor [25]. Although a pivotal trial to prove its effectiveness is lacking, nonabsorbable disaccharides continue to be recommended as the first-line therapy because of decades of clinical experience supporting its effectiveness [26].

Rifaximin

Rifaximin is a rifampicin derivative and is mostly unabsorbed by the intestine. Rifaximin is Food and Drug Administration (FDA) approved only for prevention of recurrent HE based on a large multicenter randomized trial [27]. Interestingly, it was not effective in preventing HE in a setting of a transjugular intrahe-patic portosystemic shunt (TIPS) [28]. For treating episodic overt HE, the data suggests that rifaximin has equivalent effi-cacy compared to nonabsorbable disaccharides [29–31]. Although rifaximin is better tolerated in most studies compared to lactulose, the question of using rifaximin as monotherapy for overt HE remains unanswered given the small number of trials. The use of rifaximin in addition to lactulose for overt HE is supported by a randomized controlled trial (RCT) that found a higher proportion of HE reversal in rifaximin and lactulose group compared to lactulose and placebo group (76% vs. 50.8%, $P < 0.004$) in patients with overt HE [32]. This study also reported a significant decrease in mortality in the rifaximin and lactulose group compared to lactulose and placebo group (23.8% vs. 49.1%, $P < 0.05$). However, the generalizability of this finding is limited because of the higher-than-expected mortality rate observed in the control arm (49.1%) when compared to the reported inpatient mortality due to HE in the United States (15%) [4, 33].

Neomycin, Metronidazole, and Vancomycin

Neomycin is a poorly absorbed aminoglycoside. It is used to decrease gut bacteria-derived ammonia and it is approved by FDA for use in episodic overt HE but not chronic HE. Earlier RCTs did not find difference in its efficacy when compared to lactulose [34] or placebo [35]. Neomycin was widely used in the past. However, the evidence for neomycin in episodic overt HE is weak, and its use is complicated by the risk of ototoxicity and nephrotoxicity. There are small trials supporting the short-term use of metronidazole and vancomycin [36, 37]. However, the risk of neurotoxicity and vancomycin-resistant enterococci colonization limit its long-term use.

Zinc

Zinc is important in ammonia reduction pathways both for ammonia conversion to urea in liver and for ammonia conversion to glutamine in skeletal muscle. Zinc deficiency is very common in cirrhosis. Zinc supplement has been shown to increase the speed of urea formation from ammonia and amino acid [38]. Data to support zinc use are very limited and the results are mixed. Furthermore, previous RCTs ($n = 15$–90) included chronic HE in the study, thus limiting the generalizability in episodic HE setting [39–41]. The most recent RCT of 79 patients with overt HE showed that zinc supplement was effective in deceasing HE grade and blood ammonia levels [42].

This is the only recent study with evidence to support the use of zinc in HE. The optimal dose of zinc supplement remains unknown.

ʟ-Ornithine ʟ-Aspartate

ʟ-Ornithine ʟ-aspartate (LOLA) is not available in the United States, but it is frequently used for HE treatment outside the United States. The mechanism of LOLA is to increase ammonia reduction in both liver and skeletal muscle. In the liver, LOLA can increase urea formation by stimulating ornithine transcarbamolyase and carbamoyl phosphate synthetase. In skeletal muscle, LOLA can stimulate glutamine synthesis. Data to support the use of LOLA are mainly in the setting of chronic HE and the efficacy of LOLA in episodic overt HE is not validated [43, 44]. One study from Pakistan evaluated LOLA as adjunctive treatment versus placebo in patients with episodic overt HE and found higher improvement rate of HE grade 2 in LOLA compared to placebo group [45].

Branched-Chain Amino Acids

Branched-chain amino acids (BCAAs) consist of valine, leucine, and isoleucine. In skeletal muscle, BCAAs are the substrate for glutamate which is used to synthesize glutamine in ammonia detoxification. The decrease in BCAA level and the increase in aromatic acids have been observed in cirrhosis and hepatic encephalopathy [46]. Studies have evaluated the effects of BCAAs, either intravenously or orally. For cirrhotic patients, two RCTs found that BCAAs improved important composite end points of death/hospitalization metrics in one study [47] and hepatic failure, variceal bleeding, hepatocellular carcinoma, and mortality in a second study [48]. In the recent meta-analysis of 16 RCTs with 827 patients with hepatic encephalopathy [49],

BCAAs had a beneficial effect on hepatic encephalopathy (RR 0.76, 95% CI 0.63–0.92) but there was no difference in mortality (RR 0.88, 95% CI 0.69–1.11). Currently, the European Society for Parenteral and Enteral Nutrition (ESPEN) guideline provides a grade A recommendation for the use of BCAA-enriched enteral formula in patients with hepatic encephalopathy who require enteral nutrition [50]. For parenteral nutrition, ESPEN guideline provides a grade A recommendation for the use of BCAAs in hepatic encephalopathy grades 3 and 4 [51].

Percutaneous Embolization of Large Portosystemic Shunts

Patients with large portosystemic shunts usually present with persistent HE resulting in episodic hospital admission and coma. In some patients with HE, large portosystemic shunts are accessible to embolization. Multiple retrospective studies have reported the efficacy and safety of the embolization of large portosystemic shunts in refractory HE [52–55]. In a European multicenter study ($n = 37$), 59% and 49% were free of HE at 100 days and 2 years, respectively. The HE recurrence was less in those with MELD score of 11 or less [52]. In a US series ($n = 20$), 100% (20/20) achieved immediate improvement and durable benefit was achieved in 92% (11/12) at 6–12 months after the procedure [55]. The overall procedural complication rate was 10%. One patient had bacterial cholangitis and another patient required readmission from pain at the puncture site. Importantly, 35% (7/20) developed evidence of worsening portal hypertension at some point within 12-month follow-up time [55]. In a Korean case-control series ($n = 17$), the 2-year HE recurrence rate was lower in the embolization group (40% vs. 80%, $P = 0.02$) but there was no difference in the 2-year overall survival rates (65% vs. 53%, $P = 0.98$). In addition, they observed an improvement in overall survival in the embolization group (100% vs. 60%, $P = 0.03$) in the subgroup analysis of only patients without hepatocellular carcinoma and with MELD score < 15 [54].

Molecular Adsorbent Recirculating System

Albumin has been shown to be a multifunctional protein with antioxidant, immunomodulatory, and detoxification functions [56]. Molecular adsorbent recirculating system (MARS) was introduced in 1999 and is based on the concept of albumin dialysis. MARS was designed to remove protein- and albumin-bound toxins, such as bilirubin, bile acids, nitrous oxide, and endogenous benzodiazepines. In addition, MARS also removes non-protein-bound ammonia that accumulates in liver failure [57]. Although there was no survival benefit observed in previous trials, MARS did show a beneficial effect on HE treatment. In a study designed specifically to evaluate the effect of MARS on HE, 70 patients with grade 3–4 HE were enrolled. The MARS-treated patients were found to have a higher proportion of patients with a 2-grade improvement in HE when compared to standard treatment alone. The MARS-treated patients were also found to have more rapid improvement [58]. The RELIEF trial enrolled 189 patients with ACLF and showed higher proportion of patients with HE grade 3 or 4 improvement to HE grade 0 or 1 in MARS-treated patients (15 of 24; 62.5%) compared with standard therapy (13 of 34; 38.2%), which trended toward significance ($P = 0.07$) [59]. In a small study, MARS had a statistically significant effect on improvement of HE in nine patients with alcoholic hepatitis and HE [60]. The FDA initially approved the use of MARS for grade 3–4 HE related to decompensation of chronic liver disease but has since retracted its approval. In summary, MARS is a reasonable option for patients with severe HE refractory to standard medical therapy.

Liver Transplantation

Liver transplantation (LT) is the most definitive treatment option for HE. Therefore, cirrhotic patients with HE and MELD ≥15 should be evaluated for liver transplantation. It is important to distinguish other conditions such as neurodegenerative diseases like Alzheimer's, and Wernicke's encephalopathy, which would not improve after liver transplant. Although HE should improve after LT, pretransplant episodes of HE are associated with impair of posttransplant neurological outcome [61]. Data are limited for liver transplant outcomes in patients with HE in the setting of ACLF. Although posttransplant survival rates for ACLF have been reported to be 80–90%, long-term outcome is scarce [10]. Patients with ACLF usually have high MELD scores but they may have LT contraindication such as active infection, and hemodynamic instability with the need for inotropes.

With the current organ allocation system using the MELDNa score, HE does not result in a higher prioritization for LT. However, there are cases with severe HE who would benefit from LT, particularly in the context of ACLF. A new scoring system, chronic liver failure consortium ACLF score (CLIF-C ACLFs), has been developed and validated in cirrhotic patients with ACLF. This score will need further evaluation to determine whether it can accurately discriminate or rank individuals according to their mortality risk, before it could be utilized for organ allocation in ACLF setting [62].

References

1. Amodio P, Del Piccolo F, Petteno E, et al. Prevalence and prognostic value of quantified electroencephalogram (EEG) alterations in cirrhotic patients. J Hepatol. 2001;35(1):37–45.

2. Romero-Gómez M, Boza F, García-Valdecasas MS, García E, Aguilar-Reina J. Subclinical hepatic encephalopathy predicts the development of overt hepatic encephalopathy. Am J Gastroenterol. 2001;96(9):2718–23.
3. Boyer TD, Haskal ZJ, American Association for the Study of Liver Diseases. The role of transjugular intrahepatic portosystemic shunt in the management of portal hypertension. Hepatology. 2005;41(2):386–400.
4. Stepanova M, Mishra A, Venkatesan C, Younossi ZM. In-hospital mortality and economic burden associated with hepatic encephalopathy in the United States from 2005 to 2009. Clin Gastroenterol Hepatol. 2012;10(9):1034–1041.e1031.
5. Stewart CA, Malinchoc M, Kim WR, Kamath PS. Hepatic encephalopathy as a predictor of survival in patients with end-stage liver disease. Liver Transplant. 2007;13(10):1366–71.
6. Bajaj JS, O'Leary JG, Tandon P, et al. Hepatic encephalopathy is associated with mortality in patients with cirrhosis independent of other extrahepatic organ failures. Clin Gastroenterol Hepatol. 2017;15(4):565–574.e564.
7. Asrani SK, Simonetto DA, Kamath PS. Acute-on-chronic liver failure. Clin Gastroenterol Hepatol. 2015;13(12):2128–39.
8. Moreau R, Jalan R, Gines P. et al. Acute-on-chronic liver failure is a distinct syndrome that develops in patients with acute decompensation of cirrhosis. Gastroenterology. 2013;144(7):1426–37. 1437.e1421–9
9. Bajaj JS, O'Leary JG, Reddy KR, et al. Survival in infection-related acute-on-chronic liver failure is defined by extrahepatic organ failures. Hepatology. 2014;60(1):250–6.
10. Sarin SK, Kumar A, Almeida JA, et al. Acute-on-chronic liver failure: consensus recommendations of the Asian Pacific association for the study of the liver (APASL). Hepatol Int. 2008;3(1):269.
11. Jalan R, Yurdaydin C, Bajaj JS, et al. Toward an improved definition of acute-on-chronic liver failure. Gastroenterology. 2014;147(1):4–10.
12. Allen AM, Kim WR, Moriarty JP, Shah ND, Larson JJ, Kamath PS. Time trends in the health care burden and mortality of acute on chronic liver failure in the United States. Hepatology. 2016;64(6):2165–72.
13. Fichet J, Mercier E, Genee O, et al. Prognosis and 1-year mortality of intensive care unit patients with severe hepatic encephalopathy. J Crit Care. 2009;24(3):364–70.
14. Cordoba J, Ventura-Cots M, Simon-Talero M, et al. Characteristics, risk factors, and mortality of cirrhotic patients hospitalized for

hepatic encephalopathy with and without acute-on-chronic liver failure (ACLF). J Hepatol. 2014;60(2):275–81.

15. Shawcross DL, Davies NA, Williams R, Jalan R. Systemic inflammatory response exacerbates the neuropsychological effects of induced hyperammonemia in cirrhosis. J Hepatol. 2004;40(2):247–54.

16. Jalan R, Gines P, Olson JC, et al. Acute-on chronic liver failure. J Hepatol. 2012;57(6):1336–48.

17. Jaeschke H. Reactive oxygen and mechanisms of inflammatory liver injury: present concepts. J Gastroenterol Hepatol. 2011;26(Suppl 1):173–9.

18. Kubes P, Mehal WZ. Sterile inflammation in the liver. Gastroenterology. 2012;143(5):1158–72.

19. Bosoi CR, Parent-Robitaille C, Anderson K, Tremblay M, Rose CF. AST-120 (spherical carbon adsorbent) lowers ammonia levels and attenuates brain edema in bile duct-ligated rats. Hepatology. 2011;53(6):1995–2002.

20. Wright G, Vairappan B, Stadlbauer V, Mookerjee RP, Davies NA, Jalan R. Reduction in hyperammonaemia by ornithine phenylacetate prevents lipopolysaccharide-induced brain edema and coma in cirrhotic rats. Liver Int. 2012;32(3):410–9.

21. Joshi D, O'Grady J, Patel A, et al. Cerebral oedema is rare in acute-on-chronic liver failure patients presenting with high-grade hepatic encephalopathy. Liver Int. 2014;34(3):362–6.

22. Nath K, Saraswat VA, Krishna YR, et al. Quantification of cerebral edema on diffusion tensor imaging in acute-on-chronic liver failure. NMR Biomed. 2008;21(7):713–22.

23. Wright G, Davies NA, Shawcross DL, et al. Endotoxemia produces coma and brain swelling in bile duct ligated rats. Hepatology. 2007;45(6):1517–26.

24. Als-Nielsen B, Gluud LL, Gluud C. Non-absorbable disaccharides for hepatic encephalopathy: systematic review of randomised trials. BMJ. 2004;328(7447):1046.

25. Leise MD, Kim WR. Rifaximin in hepatic encephalopathy: is an ounce of prevention worth a pretty penny? Gastroenterology. 2010;139(4):1416–8.

26. Vilstrup H, Amodio P, Bajaj J, et al. Hepatic encephalopathy in chronic liver disease: 2014 Practice Guideline by the American Association for the Study of Liver Diseases and the European Association for the Study of the Liver. Hepatology. 2014;60(2):715–35.

27. Bass NM, Mullen KD, Sanyal A, et al. Rifaximin treatment in hepatic encephalopathy. N Engl J Med. 2010;362(12):1071–81.
28. Riggio O, Masini A, Efrati C, et al. Pharmacological prophylaxis of hepatic encephalopathy after transjugular intrahepatic portosystemic shunt: a randomized controlled study. J Hepatol. 2005;42(5):674–9.
29. Mas A, Rodes J, Sunyer L, et al. Comparison of rifaximin and lactitol in the treatment of acute hepatic encephalopathy: results of a randomized, double-blind, double-dummy, controlled clinical trial. J Hepatol. 2003;38(1):51–8.
30. Paik YH, Lee KS, Han KH, et al. Comparison of rifaximin and lactulose for the treatment of hepatic encephalopathy: a prospective randomized study. Yonsei Med J. 2005;46(3):399–407.
31. Jiang Q, Jiang XH, Zheng MH, Jiang LM, Chen YP, Wang L. Rifaximin versus nonabsorbable disaccharides in the management of hepatic encephalopathy: a meta-analysis. Eur J Gastroenterol Hepatol. 2008;20(11):1064–70.
32. Sharma BC, Sharma P, Lunia MK, Srivastava S, Goyal R, Sarin SK. A randomized, double-blind, controlled trial comparing rifaximin plus lactulose with lactulose alone in treatment of overt hepatic encephalopathy. Am J Gastroenterol. 2013;108(9):1458–63.
33. Congly SE, Leise MD. Rifaximin for episodic, overt hepatic encephalopathy: the data are catching up to clinical practice, but questions remain. Am J Gastroenterol. 2014;109(4):598.
34. Atterbury CE, Maddrey WC, Conn HO. Neomycin-sorbitol and lactulose in the treatment of acute portal-systemic encephalopathy. A controlled, double-blind clinical trial. Am J Dig Dis. 1978;23(5):398–406.
35. Strauss E, Tramote R, Silva EP, et al. Double-blind randomized clinical trial comparing neomycin and placebo in the treatment of exogenous hepatic encephalopathy. Hepato-Gastroenterology. 1992;39(6):542–5.
36. Tarao K, Ikeda T, Hayashi K, et al. Successful use of vancomycin hydrochloride in the treatment of lactulose resistant chronic hepatic encephalopathy. Gut. 1990;31(6):702–6.
37. Morgan MH, Read AE, Speller DC. Treatment of hepatic encephalopathy with metronidazole. Gut. 1982;23(1):1–7.
38. Marchesini G, Fabbri A, Bianchi G, Brizi M, Zoli M. Zinc supplementation and amino acid-nitrogen metabolism in patients with advanced cirrhosis. Hepatology. 1996;23(5):1084–92.

39. Bresci G, Parisi G, Banti S. Management of hepatic encephalopathy with oral zinc supplementation: a long-term treatment. Eur J Med. 1993;2(7):414–6.
40. Reding P, Duchateau J, Bataille C. Oral zinc supplementation improves hepatic encephalopathy. Results of a randomised controlled trial. Lancet. 1984;2(8401):493–5.
41. Riggio O, Ariosto F, Merli M, et al. Short-term oral zinc supplementation does not improve chronic hepatic encephalopathy. Dig Dis Sci. 1991;36(9):1204–8.
42. Takuma Y, Nouso K, Makino Y, Hayashi M, Takahashi H. Clinical trial: oral zinc in hepatic encephalopathy. Aliment Pharmacol Ther. 2010;32(9):1080–90.
43. Kircheis G, Nilius R, Held C, et al. Therapeutic efficacy of L-ornithine-L-aspartate infusions in patients with cirrhosis and hepatic encephalopathy: results of a placebo-controlled, double-blind study. Hepatology. 1997;25(6):1351–60.
44. Stauch S, Kircheis G, Adler G, et al. Oral L-ornithine-L-aspartate therapy of chronic hepatic encephalopathy: results of a placebo-controlled double-blind study. J Hepatol. 1998;28(5):856–64.
45. Abid S, Jafri W, Mumtaz K, et al. Efficacy of L-ornithine-L-aspartate as an adjuvant therapy in cirrhotic patients with hepatic encephalopathy. J Coll Physicians Surg Pak. 2011;21(11):666–71.
46. Kawaguchi T, Izumi N, Charlton MR, Sata M. Branched-chain amino acids as pharmacological nutrients in chronic liver disease. Hepatology. 2011;54(3):1063–70.
47. Marchesini G, Bianchi G, Merli M, et al. Nutritional supplementation with branched-chain amino acids in advanced cirrhosis: a double-blind, randomized trial. Gastroenterology. 2003;124(7):1792–801.
48. Muto Y, Sato S, Watanabe A, et al. Effects of oral branched-chain amino acid granules on event-free survival in patients with liver cirrhosis. Clin Gastroenterol Hepatol. 2005;3(7):705–13.
49. Gluud LL, Dam G, Les I, et al. Branched-chain amino acids for people with hepatic encephalopathy. Cochrane Database Syst Rev. 2017;5:Cd001939.
50. Plauth M, Cabre E, Riggio O, et al. ESPEN guidelines on enteral nutrition: liver disease. Clin Nutr. 2006;25(2):285–94.
51. Plauth M, Cabre E, Campillo B, et al. ESPEN guidelines on parenteral nutrition: hepatology. Clin Nutr. 2009;28(4):436–44.
52. Laleman W, Simon-Talero M, Maleux G, et al. Embolization of large spontaneous portosystemic shunts for refractory hepatic encepha-

lopathy: a multicenter survey on safety and efficacy. Hepatology. 2013;57(6):2448–57.

53. Singh S, Kamath PS, Andrews JC, Leise MD. Embolization of spontaneous portosystemic shunts for management of severe persistent hepatic encephalopathy. Hepatology. 2014;59(2):735–6.

54. An J, Kim KW, Han S, Lee J, Lim YS. Improvement in survival associated with embolisation of spontaneous portosystemic shunt in patients with recurrent hepatic encephalopathy. Aliment Pharmacol Ther. 2014;39(12):1418–26.

55. Lynn AM, Singh S, Congly SE, et al. Embolization of portosystemic shunts for treatment of medically refractory hepatic encephalopathy. Liver Transplant. 2016;22(6):723–31.

56. Garcia-Martinez R, Caraceni P, Bernardi M, Gines P, Arroyo V, Jalan R. Albumin: pathophysiologic basis of its role in the treatment of cirrhosis and its complications. Hepatology. 2013;58(5):1836–46.

57. Leise MD, Poterucha JJ, Kamath PS, Kim WR. Management of hepatic encephalopathy in the hospital. Mayo Clin Proc. 2014;89(2):241–53.

58. Hassanein TI, Tofteng F, Brown RS Jr, et al. Randomized controlled study of extracorporeal albumin dialysis for hepatic encephalopathy in advanced cirrhosis. Hepatology. 2007;46(6):1853–62.

59. Banares R, Nevens F, Larsen FS, et al. Extracorporeal albumin dialysis with the molecular adsorbent recirculating system in acute-on-chronic liver failure: the RELIEF trial. Hepatology. 2013;57(3):1153–62.

60. Pares A, Deulofeu R, Cisneros L, et al. Albumin dialysis improves hepatic encephalopathy and decreases circulating phenolic aromatic amino acids in patients with alcoholic hepatitis and severe liver failure. Crit Care. 2009;13(1):R8.

61. Garcia-Martinez R, Rovira A, Alonso J, et al. Hepatic encephalopathy is associated with posttransplant cognitive function and brain volume. Liver Transplant. 2011;17(1):38–46.

62. Jalan R, Saliba F, Pavesi M, et al. Development and validation of a prognostic score to predict mortality in patients with acute-on-chronic liver failure. J Hepatol. 2014;61(5):1038–47.

Chapter 7
Prevention of Recurrence of Hepatic Encephalopathy

Sudhir Maharshi and Barjesh Chander Sharma

Introduction

Hepatic encephalopathy (HE) is a neuropsychiatric syndrome defined by symptoms manifested in a continuum, as deterioration in mental state, with psychomotor dysfunction, increased reaction time, impaired memory, poor concentration, disorientation, sensory abnormalities, and in severe form—coma [1–3]. Recurrence of HE is seen in 47–57% of patients at the end of 1 year. Occurrence of each episode of HE is associated with increased morbidity, hospitalization, healthcare burden, poor prognosis, and increased mortality [4–6]. Overt HE is observed in 30–45% of patients with chronic liver disease and 10–50% of patients with a transjugular intrahepatic portosystemic shunt (TIPS) while minimal hepatic encephalopathy (MHE) affects 20–60% of patients with liver cirrhosis [7].

S. Maharshi, M.B.B.S., D.N.B., D.M.
Department of Gastroenterology, SMS Medical College,
Jaipur, India

B. C. Sharma, M.D., D.M. (✉)
Department of Gastroenterology, G.B. Pant Hospital,
New Delhi, India

© Springer International Publishing AG, part of Springer Nature 2018   99
J. S. Bajaj (ed.), *Diagnosis and Management of Hepatic
Encephalopathy*, https://doi.org/10.1007/978-3-319-76798-7_7

Primary prophylaxis is defined as treating the patients to prevent development of first episode of HE and secondary prophylaxis is preventing recurrence of HE in patients who had a previous episode of HE.

Case-1: A 48-year-old male, case of alcoholic cirrhosis Child class C with portal hypertension decompensated with ascites, HE, and variceal bleed, was admitted 1 month back in our hospital with HE. He was treated at that time with lactulose and other supportive treatment. He was readmitted 2 days back with overt HE. What are the available treatment options in this patient with recurrent HE?

Treatment for secondary prophylaxis or prevention of recurrence of HE can be classified as follows: luminal agents, extraluminal agents, and interventions [7] (Table 7.1).

1. Luminal agents—This category includes drugs that act by reducing the nitrogenous load in the gut in patients with impaired liver function and portosystemic shunting like non-absorbable disaccharides lactulose and lactitol, rifaximin, and probiotics [4–6].
2. Extraluminal agents—This category includes drugs that reduce ammonia by providing alternative pathways of metabolism like branched-chain amino acids (BCAA) and glycerol phenylbutyrate (GBP).
3. Interventions—This category includes interventions that decrease portosystemic shunting by embolization of large spontaneous shunts or balloon-occluded retrograde transvenous obliteration (BRTO) of large spontaneous splenorenal shunts [8–11].

Table 7.1 Studies of therapy for the prevention of recurrence of HE

Study	Study design	Dose and duration of drugs	Results
Sharma et al. (2009) [4]	Open-label RCT Cirrhotic patients, recovered from HE	HE—L (n = 70): Lactulose HE—NL (n = 70): No lactulose Lactulose dose 30–60 mL/day in two or three divided doses Duration 6 months	Over median follow-up 14 months HE developed in 19.6% patients in HE-L vs. 46.8% in HE-NL group (P = 0.001)
Bass et al. (2010) [5]	Double-blind RCT Cirrhotic patients, recurrent HE (at least two HE episodes in past 6 months)	Rifaximin (n = 140): 550 mg two times/day Placebo (n = 159) ~90% patients received lactulose (average daily dose ~30 g) Duration 6 months or until therapy was discontinued	First breakthrough HE episode: 22.1% in rifaximin group vs. 45.9% in placebo group (HR 0.42, 95% CI 0.28–0.64; P < 0.001)
Sanyal et al. (2011)[14]	Parallel study with study by Bass et al. (2010) [5]		CLDQ scores: significantly higher with rifaximin vs. placebo (P < 0.05) Remission maintained: 74.2% with rifaximin vs. 50% with placebo

(continued)

Table 7.1 (continued)

Study	Study design	Dose and duration of drugs	Results
Agrawal et al. (2012) [6]	Open-label RCT Cirrhotic patients, recovered from HE	Group L ($n = 80$): Lactulose Group P ($n = 77$): Probiotics Group N ($n = 78$): No therapy Lactulose dose 30–60 mL/day Probiotics 112.5 billion viable lyophilized bacteria per capsule Duration 12 months	At the end of study the proportion of patients with HE was less in the lactulose and probiotic group than in the no-therapy group (26.5% vs. 34.4% vs. 56.9%, $P = 0.001$)
Dhiman et al. (2014) [20]	Double-blind RCT Cirrhotic patients, recovered from HE	Probiotic group ($n = 66$): VSL#3 sachet, 9×10^{11} bacteria daily Placebo ($n = 64$): corn flour placebo sachet daily Duration 6 months	Breakthrough HE episode: 34.8% in probiotic group vs. 51.6% in placebo group (HR 0.65, 95% CI 0.38–1.11; $P = 0.12$)
Rockey et al. (2014) [8]	Double blind RCT Cirrhotic patients, ≥2 HE episode in previous 6 months	GPB group ($n = 90$): glycerol phenylbutyrate (GPB) 6 mL twice daily Placebo ($n = 88$): Placebo 6 mL twice daily 59 patients were already on rifaximin Duration 16 weeks	Proportion of patients who experienced an HE event: 21% in GPB group vs. 36% in placebo group; $P = 0.02$

Table 7.1 (continued)

Study	Study design	Dose and duration of drugs	Results
Les et al. (2011) [9]	Double-blind RCT Cirrhotic patients, one HE episode in previous 2 months	BCAA group (n = 58): BCAA supplement 30 g white powder (leucine −13.5 g, isoleucine—9 g, valine 7.5 g) MDX group (n = 58): Maltodextrin (MDX) supplement Duration 56 weeks	Actuarial risk of remaining free of HE: 47% in BCAA group vs. 34% in MDX group; $P = 0.274$
Mukund et al. (2012) [11]	Retrospective analysis Cirrhotic patients with recurrent HE with large portosystemic shunt	Eight session of BRTO with sodium tetradecyl sulfate foam performed in seven patient	Improvement in HE was seen within 48 h of procedure in six of the seven patients (86%) and at the end of 4 months HE was completely resolved in these patients

(continued)

Table 7.1 (continued)

Study	Study design	Dose and duration of drugs	Results
Laleman et al. (2013) [10]	Retrospective cohort study Cirrhotic patients and chronic refractory HE with large spontaneous portosystemic shunts (SPSSs)	$N = 37$ patients who underwent embolization (performed using coil, amplatzer plugs, or matrix or a combination of these)	On a short-term basis (i.e., within 100 days after embolization) 59.4% were free of HE ($P < 0.001$ vs. before embolization) 48.6% of patients remained HE free over a mean follow-up period of 697 ± 157 days ($P < 0.001$ vs. before embolization)
Bajaj et al. (2017) [23]	Open-label RCT Cirrhotic patients with recurrent HE	Group 1: FMT using a rationally derived stool donor Group 2: Standard of care Duration 150 days	No participant developed further episode of HE in group 1 compared to five patients in group 2; $P = 0.03$

RCT randomized controlled trial, *HE* hepatic encephalopathy, *L* lactulose, *NL* no lactulose, *CLDQ* chronic liver disease questionnaire, *HE* hepatic encephalopathy, *BRTO* balloon-occluded retrograde transvenous obliteration, *BCAA* branched-chain amino acids, *SPSSs* spontaneous portosystemic shunts, *FMT* fecal microbiota transplantation

Luminal Agents

Nonabsorbable Disaccharides

Lactulose and lactitol are available nonabsorbable disaccharides used for the treatment of HE. They decrease the absorption of ammonia through a cathartic effect and by altering colonic pH. They are also effective in prevention of recurrence of HE. In a study, 125 patients who had recovered from a recent episode of HE were randomized to receive either lactulose or no lactulose for 20 months. 19.6% of patients in the lactulose group developed recurrence of HE compared to 46.8% in the no-lactulose group over a median follow-up period of 14 months (Fig. 7.1) [4]. Lactulose and probiotics

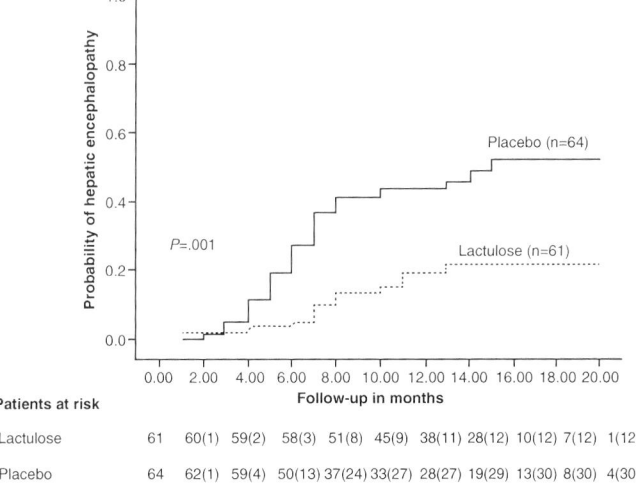

Fig. 7.1 Probability of developing hepatic encephalopathy (HE) in patients receiving lactulose (dotted line) or placebo (continuous line). Figures in parentheses indicate the cumulative number of subjects who developed HE (with permission from Gastroenterology 2009;137:885–91)

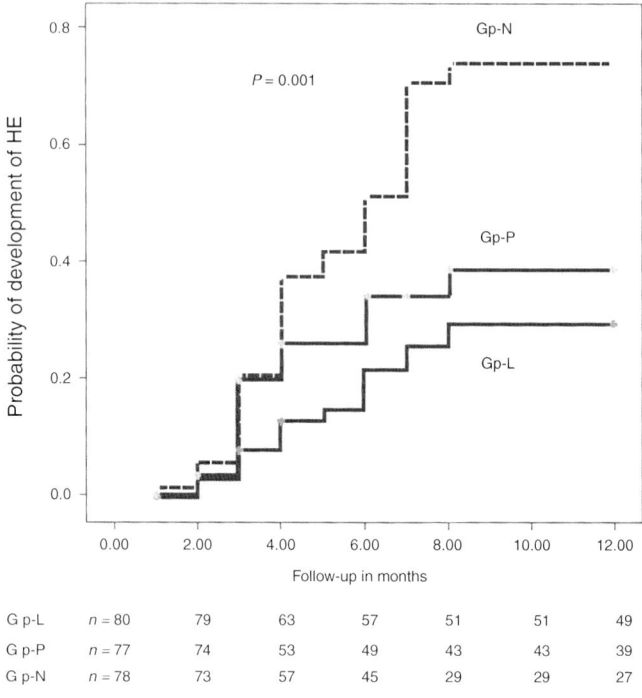

Fig. 7.2 Probability of developing hepatic encephalopathy in patients receiving lactulose (Gp-L), probiotic treatment (Gp-P), or no therapy (Gp-N) (with permission from Am J Gastroenterol 2012;107:1043–50)

were equally effective in another study for secondary prophylaxis of HE compared to patients with no therapy (26.5% vs. 34.4% vs. 56.9%, $P = 0.001$) (Fig. 7.2) [6]. Nonabsorbable disaccharide therapy has certain side effects like pain abdomen, bloating, flatulence, and diarrhea which may result in noncompliance in some patients [12, 13].

Rifaximin

Rifaximin is a gut-selective, oral antimicrobial agent that is concentrated in the gastrointestinal tract and has broad-spectrum activity against gram-positive, gram-negative aerobic and anaerobic enteric bacteria, and has a low risk of bacterial resistance. Besides this, due to minimal systemic bioavailability, rifaximin may be more conducive to long-term use than other, more bioavailable antibiotics with serious side effects [5]. For prevention of recurrence of HE, a study compared rifaximin ($n = 140$) versus placebo ($n = 159$). Rifaximin or placebo was given for 6 months, or until treatment was discontinued before that time. Patients on rifaximin compared to placebo had significantly lower first breakthrough HE episodes (45.9% vs. 22.1%, $P = <0.001$) and first HE-related hospitalization (22.6% vs. 13.6%, $P = 0.01$). Adverse drug reactions and mortality were similar in both the groups [5]. Another study revealed that patients on rifaximin had significant improvement in health-related quality of life (HRQOL) compared to the placebo group [14]. Chronic liver disease questionnaire (CLDQ) score used to measure HRQOL was significantly low in patients with breakthrough HE. HRQOL significantly improved in patients who received rifaximin in combination with lactulose and worsening HRQOL may predict HE event irrespective of treatment [14]. Long-term (>24 months) therapy with rifaximin appears to provide a continued reduction in the rate of HE-related and all-cause hospitalizations, without an increased rate of drug-related adverse effects [15]. Patients on rifaximin had less frequent adverse effects and hospitalizations compared to patients on lactulose [12, 13]. A recently published study showed that there was no difference in the efficacy of traditional rifaximin dosing (400 mg three times daily) compared to newer dosing (550 mg twice daily) for the prevention of recurrence of HE. However the 550 mg regimen had a lower acquisition cost [16].

In a randomized controlled trial Riggio et al. found that therapy with lactitol or rifaximin was not effective in the prophylaxis of HE during the first months after TIPS [17].

Probiotics

Probiotics alter the gut flora with non-urease-producing organisms, resulting in a decrease in ammonia production and absorption due to a reduction in intraluminal pH. Probiotic therapy in patient with HE acts by decreasing ammonia absorption, decreasing bacterial urease activity in the lumen, decreasing ammonia in portal blood, decreasing intestinal pH, and improving the nutritional status of gut epithelium leading to decreased intestinal permeability and decreased inflammation and oxidative stress in the hepatocyte resulting in increased hepatic clearance of ammonia [18, 19]. Probiotics for HE can be used as long-term therapy with no adverse effects. In a study 235 patients who had recovered from a recent episode of HE were randomized to receive lactulose, probiotics, or no therapy for 12 months. The proportion of cirrhotic patients with HE episodes were less in the lactulose and probiotic groups compared to no-therapy group (26.5% vs. 34.4% vs. 56.9%, $P = 0.001$) (Fig. 7.2) [6]. Another study revealed trend towards reduction in development of breakthrough HE (34.8% vs. 51.6%), decreased hospitalization for HE (19.7% vs. 42.2%), and less complications of cirrhosis (24.2% vs. 45.3%) in patients treated with probiotics compared to placebo [20]. The probiotic preparation used in this study was VSL#3®, and contains four *Lactobacillus* spp. (*L. paracasei*, *L. plantarum*, *L. acidophilus,* and *L. delbrueckii* subsp. *bulgaricus*), three *Bifidobacterium* spp. (*B. longum, B. infantis,* and *B. breve*), and *Streptococcus thermophilus.* This preparation is formulated as a granulated powder (20 mesh) of 9×10^{11} colony-forming units per sachet in defined ratios of lyophilized bacteria.

Extraluminal Agents

Glycerol Phenylbutyrate

Glycerol phenylbutyrate (GPB) consists of three molecules of phenylbutyric acid joined to glycerol by ester linkage and is odorless and tasteless liquid that lowers ammonia by providing an alternate pathway to urea for waste nitrogen excretion in the form of phenylacetyl glutamine, which is excreted in urine. GPB 6 mL orally twice daily significantly reduced recurrence of HE (21% vs. 36%; $P = 0.02$), time to first event (hazard ratio [HR] = 0.56; $P < 0.05$), and total events (35 vs. 57; $P = 0.04$), and was associated with fewer HE-related hospitalizations (13 vs. 25; $P = 0.06$) compared with placebo. Drug-related adverse events were similar in both the groups [8].

Branched-Chain Amino Acids (BCAA)

The plasma amino acid profile in patients with liver cirrhosis is altered with a decrease in BCAA and increase in aromatic amino acids (AAA). The BCAAs are a source of glutamate which helps to metabolize ammonia in skeletal muscle. In a recently published study, BCAA was administered to 58 patients with one previous episode of HE, and compared to 58 patients receiving maltodextrin. There was no significant difference in the frequency of recurrent HE, but BCAA improves MHE and muscle mass significantly [9].

Case-2: A 65-year-old male, case of liver cirrhosis Child class A, nonalcoholic fatty liver disease related decompensated with HE, was admitted in our hospital thrice in last 2 months with overt HE. Ultrasound abdomen with Doppler showed evidence of chronic liver disease, and dilated portal vein (16 mm) with multiple portosystemic collaterals. What are the available treatment options in such a group of patients with recurrent HE due to portosystemic shunts?

Interventions

Embolization of Large Spontaneous Shunt

Patients with refractory HE may have large spontaneous portosystemic shunts (SPSSs). Two large studies have been published demonstrating efficacy and safety of embolization of large portosystemic shunts in patient with recurrent HE. In the European multicenter cohort study ($n = 37$), 59% of patients were free of HE within 100 days and 48% were free of HE over a mean follow-up period of 697 ± 157 days [10]. In this study one patient developed hepatic capsular hemorrhage; otherwise there were no other major periprocedural complications. Long-term safety appeared good with no increase in variceal bleeding. In another study ($n = 15$), 90% of cirrhotics improved at 2 months post-procedure [21]. One patient developed an infected hepatic cyst 2 weeks post-procedure; otherwise there were no significant complications related to the procedure. The median MELD score in both the studies was 13. Logistic regression performed in the European study suggested that patients with MELD score > 11 were at risk of HE recurrence after shunt embolization.

Balloon-Occluded Retrograde Transvenous Obliteration

Treatment with BRTO in patients with severe recurrent HE with large spontaneous splenorenal shunt revealed clinical improvement of HE in 86% patients with decrease in arterial ammonia levels while one patient showed delayed improvement [11].

Case-3: A 54-year-old male, case of liver cirrhosis Child class C, HCV-related portal hypertension decompensated with ascites, HE, and hepatorenal syndrome, underwent TIPS 3 weeks back for refractory ascites. Presently he is admitted with frequent episode of overt HE. What are the treatment options for this patient?

Recurrent HE in post-TIPS patients may ameliorate by reducing the stent diameter or by occluding the shunt. However this may result in increased complications related to portal hypertension such as variceal bleeding and refractory ascites [10].

Case-4: A 54-year-old male, case of liver cirrhosis Child class C, HBV-related portal hypertension decompensated with ascites and HE, was admitted in our hospital twice in last 1 month with overt HE despite being on lactulose therapy for prevention of HE recurrence. What are the available treatment options in such a patient?

Patients with recurrent episodes of HE despite lactulose therapy usually benefit from the addition of rifaximin, which decreases the frequency of recurrent HE episodes and related hospitalizations [22]. Thus combination of rifaximin and lactulose may be considered for the prevention of recurrence of HE. Fecal microbiota transplantation (FMT) is also an option for prevention of HE recurrence. A recently published study showed that FMT prevents HE recurrence, and improve cognition and dysbiosis without any serious adverse events in cirrhotic patients [23]. Another study revealed that FMT enables protective effects in HE rats and it improves the cognitive functions [24]. If recurrent HE persists despite being on above therapies, option of liver transplant should be considered in patient with decompensated liver cirrhosis.

Conclusion

Prevention of recurrence of HE should be considered in each patient as recurrent episodes of HE are associated with increased healthcare burden, poor prognosis, and mortality. Nonabsorbable disaccharides, rifaximin, probiotics, GPB, and embolization of large portosystemic shunt are proven options for prevention of recurrence of HE.

Flowchart: Prevention of recurrence of hepatic encephalopathy

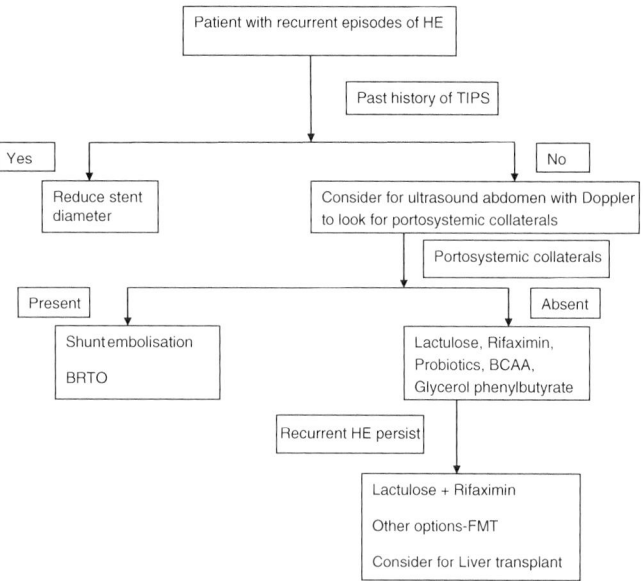

(*HE* hepatic encephalopathy, *TIPS* transjugular intrahepatic portosystemic shunt, *BRTO* balloon-occluded retrograde transvenous obliteration, *BCCA* branched-chain amino acids, *FMT* fecal microbiota transplantation)

References

1. Poordad FF. The burden of hepatic encephalopathy. Aliment Pharmacol Ther. 2007;25(suppl 1):3–9.
2. Stewart CA, Malinchoc M, Kim WR, Kamath PS. Hepatic encephalopathy as a predictor of survival in patients with end stage liver disease. Liver Transpl. 2007;13:1366–71.
3. Ferenci P, Lockwood A, Mullen K, Tarter R, Weissenborn K, Blei AT. Hepatic encephalopathy—definition, nomenclature, diagnosis and quantification: final report of the working party at the 11th World Congress of Gastroenterology, Vienna, 1998. Hepatology. 2002;35:716–21.
4. Sharma BC, Sharma P, Agrawal A, Sarin SK. Secondary prophylaxis of hepatic encephalopathy: an open-label randomized controlled trial of lactulose versus placebo. Gastroenterology. 2009;137:885–91.
5. Bass NM, Mullen KD, Sanyal A, Poordad F, Neff G, Leevy CB, et al. Rifaximin treatment in hepatic encephalopathy. N Engl J Med. 2010;362:1071–81.
6. Agrawal A, Sharma BC, Sharma P, Sarin SK. Secondary prophylaxis of hepatic encephalopathy in cirrhosis: an open-label, randomized controlled trial of lactulose, probiotics, and no therapy. Am J Gastroenterol. 2012;107(7):1043–50.
7. Sharma BC, Maharshi S. Prevention of hepatic encephalopathy recurrence. Clin Liver Dis. 2015;5(3):64–7.
8. Rocky DC, Vierling JM, Mantry P, Ghabril M, Brown RS, Alexeeva O, et al. Randomized, double-blind, controlled study of glycerol, phenylbutyrate in hepatic encephalopathy. Hepatology. 2014;59:1073–83.
9. Les L, Doval E, Martinez RG, Planas M, Cárdenas G, Gómez P, et al. Effects of branched-chain amino acids supplementation in patients with cirrhosis and a previous episode of hepatic encephalopathy: a randomized study. Am J Gastroenterol. 2011;106:1081–8.
10. Laleman W, Talero SM, Maleux G, Perez M, Ameloot K, Soriano G, et al. Embolization of large spontaneous portosystemic shunts for refractory hepatic encephalopathy: a multicenter survey on safety and efficacy. Hepatology. 2013;57:2448–57.
11. Mukund A, Rajesh S, Arora A, Patidar Y, Jain D, Sarin SK. Efficacy of balloon-occluded retrograde transvenous obliteration of large spontaneous lienorenal shunt in patients with severe recurrent hepatic encephalopathy with foam sclerotherapy: initial experience. J Vasc Interv Radiol. 2012;23:1200–6.

12. Neff G. Factors affecting compliance and persistence with treatment for hepatic encephalopathy. Pharmacotherapy. 2010;30:22S–7S.

13. Leevy CB, Phillips JA. Hospitalizations during the use of rifaximin versus lactulose for the treatment of hepatic encephalopathy. Dig Dis Sci. 2007;52:737–41.

14. Sanyal A, Younossi ZM, Bass NM, Mullen KD, Poordad F, Brown RS, et al. Randomised clinical trial: rifaximin improves health-related quality of life in cirrhotic patients with hepatic encephalopathy—a double-blind placebo controlled study. Aliment Pharmacol Ther. 2011;34:853–61.

15. Mullen KD, Sanyal AJ, Bass NM, Poordad F, Sheikh MY, Frederick RT, et al. Rifaximin is safe and well tolerated for long-term maintenance remission from overt hepatic encephalopathy. Clin Gastroenterol Hepatol. 2014;12(8):1390–7.

16. Lyon KC, Likar E, Martello JL, Regier M. Retrospective cross-sectional pilot study of rifaximin dosing for the prevention of recurrent hepatic encephalopathy. J Gastroenterol Hepatol. 2017. https://doi.org/10.1111/jgh.13759.

17. Riggio O, Masini A, Efrati C, Nicolao F, Angeloni S, Salvatori FM, et al. Pharmacological prophylaxis of hepatic encephalopathy after transjugular intrahepatic portosystemic shunt: a randomized controlled study. J Hepatol. 2005;42(5):674–9.

18. Lata J, Jurankova J, Kopakova M, Vitek P. Probiotics inn hepatology. World J Gastroenterol. 2011;17:2890–6.

19. Lunia MK, Sharma BC, Sharma P, Sachdeva S, Srivastava S. Probiotics prevent hepatic encephalopathyin patients with cirrhosis: a randomized controlled trial. Clin Gastroenterol Hepatol. 2014;12(6):1003–8.

20. Dhiman RK, Rana B, Agrawal S, Garg A, Chopra M, Thumburu KK, et al. Probiotic VSL#3 reduces liver disease severity and hospitalization in patients with cirrhosis: a randomized, controlled trial. Gastroenterology. 2014;147(6):1327–37.

21. Singh S, Kamath PS, Andrews JC, Leise MD. Embolization of spontaneous portosystemic shunts for management of severe persistent hepatic encephalopathy. Hepatology. 2014;59(2):735–6.

22. Leise MD, Poterucha JJ, Kamath PS, Kim WR. Management of hepatic encephalopathy in the hospiatal. Mayo Clin Proc. 2014;89(2):241–53.

23. Bajaj JS, Kassam Z, Fagan A, Gavis EA, Lin E, Cox IJ, et al. Fecal microbiota transplant from a rational stool donor improves hepatic encephalopathy: a randomized clinical trial. Hepatology. 2017;66(6):1727–38.
24. Wang WW, Zhang Y, Huang XB, You N, Zheng L, Jing L. Fecal microbiota transplantation prevents hepatic encephalopathy in rats with carbon tetrachloride-induced acute hepatic dysfunction. World J Gastroenterol. 2017;23(38):6983–94.

Chapter 8
Hepatic Encephalopathy Diagnosis Conundrums

Sara Montagnese and Piero Amodio

Introduction

We co-manage a dedicated clinic for the diagnosis of cognitive disturbances of medical origin, with a specific clinical and research interest in HE, within a tertiary referral hepatology centre. Therefore, we are often confronted with complex cases, which are referred to us with a view to complete/define diagnoses, to optimize treatment and/or to obtain prognostic indicators of post-transplant neuropsychiatric performance. In our clinic, each patient undergoes an evaluation by an internist/hepatologist, comprehensive neuropsychological evaluation by a dedicated neuropsychologist, an electroencephalogram (EEG), critical flicker frequency and, in selected instances, sensory and cognitive evoked potentials. Where needed, the patient is reviewed after the institution or modification of treatment and/or brain imaging or other relevant investigations, as appropriate. In this chapter, our specialist experience is utilized, by way of a number of complex and interesting cases, to draw a series of

―――――
S. Montagnese (✉) · P. Amodio, M.D.
Department of Medicine, University of Padova, Padova, Italy
e-mail: sara.montagnese@unipd.it; piero.amodio@unipd.it

© Springer International Publishing AG, part of Springer Nature 2018   117
J. S. Bajaj (ed.), *Diagnosis and Management of Hepatic Encephalopathy*, https://doi.org/10.1007/978-3-319-76798-7_8

conclusions on how to define, diagnose and exclude HE within more general clinical contexts.

Instead of HE 1: Seizure in Compensated Cirrhosis and Cerebrovascular Disease

In January 2016, an 81-year-old female with hepatitis C-related compensated cirrhosis of the liver (Child-Pugh score A6 [1], MELD 11 [2], MELD-Na 11 [3]) was admitted into hospital after a fall, with a provisional accident and emergency diagnosis of HE. Her son reported finding her on the floor, confused but awake and able to communicate, with no apparent signs of trauma. Clinical examination confirmed that the patient was slowed but able to communicate, only partly orientated in space and time, with no flapping tremor, and no obvious strength/sensitivity asymmetry on neurological examination. A lesion on the tip of her tongue was compatible with tongue biting. There were no ascites, no jaundice and no other signs of hepatic decompensation; she had no history of hepatic decompensation either. Medical history included type II diabetes on insulin, arterial hypertension, non-significant carotid atherosclerosis and an admission into the neurology ward for seizures in 2013. Such episode was not well defined and the pertinent medical documents provided were incomplete; however, the patient had been started on levetiracetam. Bloods were unremarkable with no signs of infection/inflammation, normal urinalysis, normal thyroid function tests and normal ammonia levels; levetiracetam plasma levels were at the low end of the norm. Urgent, brain CT with no contrast documented moderate cerebral and cerebellar atrophy, and small white matter lesions compatible with chronic ischemic demyelination in the centrum semiovale. Two days after admission, the EEG was normal, with a mean frequency of 9 Hz and no abnormal focal activity. Neuropsychological evaluation documented isolated memory deficits, which were felt to be compatible with mild cognitive impairment (Mini Mental State Examination (MMSE) [4] 21/30), most likely of vascular origin, rather than HE. Psychomotor speed, attention and executive function tests were substantially normal for age and level of education. Therefore, based on history, neuropsychological profile and extremely low likelihood of HE (good hepatic function, no portal-systemic shunt on ultrasound and normal ammonia levels [5]) it was concluded that the episode determining hospital admission had most likely been a seizure, within the context of cerebrovascular disease. She remained on levetiracetam and short-term neurological/EEG follow-up was negative. Some 18 months later, her cirrhosis remained compensated but her neurological status had worsened and she was in a nursing home.

Instead of HE 2: Viral Encephalitis in Decompensated Cirrhosis

In January 2011, a 78-year-old female with NASH-cirrhosis (Child-Pugh score B9, MELD 14, MELD-Na 15) was admitted into hospital with a provisional accident and emergency diagnosis of a bout of recurrent HE, most likely precipitated by infection. She had had a flulike episode, after which she had started to exhibit bizarre behaviour and restlessness (for example, she had gone out in the garden during the night to hang out the laundry). Clinical examination confirmed delirium-like psychomotor agitation: the patient was nervous, restless, only partially orientated in space/time, with no flapping tremor, no obvious strength/sensitivity asymmetry on neurological examination, and no rigor. She had non-tense ascites and was jaundiced. Her white cell count was slightly raised compared to baseline, but still within the normal range at 7200/mm^3, and her CRP was raised at 42 mg/mL (<6); her ammonia levels were abnormal at 101 μmol/L (<35). She was known in our ward and outpatient clinics for a history of recurrent HE, almost invariably precipitated by constipation and manifesting itself with lethargy, up to coma. Medical history also included overweight, diabetes on oral medication and arterial hypertension. On admission, she was treated with enemas and maintained on lactulose and rifaximin. However, her mental status did not improve; she remained agitated, at times completely disorientated and unable to recognize her relatives, occasionally requiring sedation. Urgent, brain CT with no contrast was substantially negative. Five days after admission, her EEG was slightly slowed, with a mean frequency of 7–8 Hz, and a significant amount of delta activity over the frontal-central regions of the left hemisphere (Fig. 8.1). She was unable to perform any neuropsychological test. Cerebrospinal fluid on day 7 was inconclusive. However, based on clinical evolution and EEG findings, viral encephalitis was suspected and she was put on intravenous acyclovir (400 mg b.i.d.). After a few days, her mental status had returned comparable to baseline and her EEG was only slightly slowed, with no focal delta activity. She was discharged home and continued to

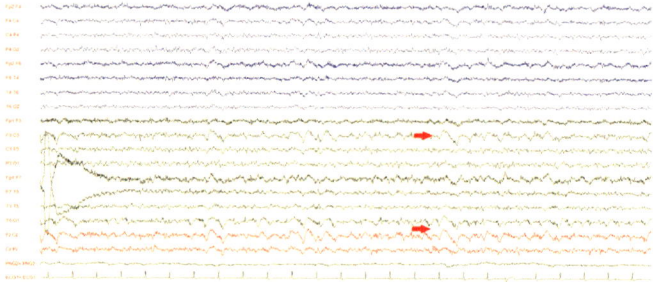

Fig. 8.1 Delta activity, with some features of pseudo-periodicity, over the frontal-central regions of the left hemisphere (red arrows) on a slightly slowed EEG (longitudinal montage; 20 s; blue = right hemisphere, front to back; black = left hemisphere, front to back, red = central areas)

be looked after in clinic for her cirrhosis, which remained stable. She died 2 years after the episode, in a different hospital, most likely of acute-on-chronic liver failure, after a fall and hip fracture.

Instead of HE 3: Cerebral Haemorrhage in Decompensated Cirrhosis

In February 2017, a 54-year-old male with decompensated alcohol-related cirrhosis was admitted into hospital for refractory ascites and transplant selection (Child-Pugh score C10, MELD 28, MELD-Na 31). He had been abstinent for 3 years and his recent medical history had been dominated by ascites, which had become very difficult to manage; he had no history of overt HE. Whilst an inpatient, he developed rapid-onset neuropsychiatric deterioration, reaching a comatose state (Glasgow Coma Scale = 6) [6] in approximately an hour, and in the absence of prior lethargy/slowing, or obvious HE precipitants. His ammonia levels were only marginally elevated at 55 µmol/L (<35), and comparable to those recorded on previous occasions both as an in- and outpatient. There were no other obvious causes for metabolic coma, with no significant abnormalities/changes in electrolytes, inflammatory makers, blood gases, urinalysis or the medication he was on. This, together with the rapid change in neurological status, was perceived as suspicious, so the doctor on call required an urgent brain CT scan. This documented a large, right frontal-parietal haemorrhagic stroke (Fig. 8.2), which opened onto the ventricular system, determining some degree of shift of the median brain structures and left lateral ventricle dilatation; uncal herniation was already present. The size of the stroke and the type of available imaging did now allow to determine whether this was a haemorrhagic stroke or an ischemic stroke with haemorrhagic transformation. The patient died approximately 10 h later.

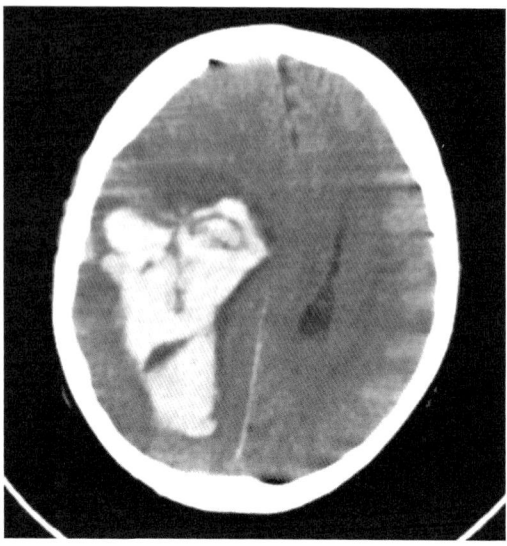

Fig. 8.2 Right frontal-parietal haemorrhagic stroke, opening onto the ventricular system and determining some degree of shift of the median brain structures, and left lateral ventricle dilatation

Together with HE 1: Alzheimer's Disease and Superimposed HE

The incidence of dementia increases with age, so in elderly patients with cirrhosis, cognitive impairment can be caused by both HE and dementia. In addition, in patients with dementia, the occurrence of HE can further deteriorate performance and behaviour. Here we describe the case of a 78-year-old female who suffered from Alzheimer's dementia (AD; MMSE 19/30) and HCV-related cirrhosis. She lived with her daughter's family. Up until 1 month prior to referral to our unit, in July 2012, she was oriented in time and space, able to walk and dress/undress, and continent. She was able to recognize relatives, and frequently remembered their names. However, she had memory problems and she was no longer allowed in the kitchen because she had burnt food and was no longer able to cook properly. She had HCV-related cirrhosis, Child-Pugh B7, MELD 11. Over the month prior to referral to our unit, her mental state had rapidly deteriorated: she was frequently disoriented in time and space, and had became unable to dress/undress herself, and unable to go to the toilet and to bed by herself. Her daughter had had to apply for a reduction in the number of her working hours, and had missed a few days' work. Rapid evolution AD or a superimposed cerebrovascular event had been suspected by her neurologist. Brain CT scan showed only brain atrophy, particularly of the hippocampus. When we examined the patient, she had MMSE 16/30, and was unable to complete the Psychometric Hepatic Encephalopathy Score (PHES) battery [7] or computerized psychometric tests. Her EEG showed theta (slow) activity in the temporal derivations. EEG slowing was confirmed on spectral analysis. Blood biochemistry documented mild anaemia (Hb = 10 g/L), low platelets 100,000, INR = 1.4, low albumin and high gamma globulins. The ammonia plasma level was elevated at 96 μmol/L (<35). An abdominal US revealed paraumbilical vein patency. Mild HE (grade could not be determined clinically because of comorbidity) superimposed to AD was suspected and lactulose (30 g b.i.d.) plus rifaximin (400 mg t.i.d.) were prescribed. Two weeks later the patient had recovered self-sufficiency, and she was oriented in space, able to dress/undress and go to the toilet and to bed by herself. MMSE was 20, the PHES score was −7 and the EEG spectral analysis still documented slow theta activity which, however, was reduced compared to the previous evaluation (40% vs. 64%). Ammonia levels had also returned within normal limits. In this instance, HE was diagnosed based on the clinical and biochemical response to ammonia-lowering treatment, despite the association with another neurological disease.

Difficult HE Diagnosis 1: An Illiterate Patient

In July 2016, a 66-year-old female with HBV-related cirrhosis (Child-Pugh score B8, MELD 14, MELD-Na 15) was referred to our outpatient unit for an extensive neuropsychological evaluation, within the context of pre-transplant workup. Her cirrhosis had never decompensated and she had no additional medical history. She was illiterate, had never gone to school and had always worked as a farmer. Lack of schooling seemed related to logistic/economic issues rather than personal/cognitive issues. She was married with two grown-up sons, one of whom had been transplanted for HBV-related cirrhosis in our unit in 2008. She was functioning well within her home and work context. Formal neuropsychiatric evaluation was complicated by the fact that besides being illiterate the patient spoke a dialect from her region in Southern Italy and had difficulties understanding instructions imparted in Italian. However, she had an extremely positive attitude towards the tests. Her EEG was completely normal with a background frequency of 11–12 Hz; PHES could not be administered because of difficulties with both letters and numbers, and a general lack of familiarity with writing and drawing. The patient had never used a computer but was more than happy and interested in trying a reaction time test, and became progressively faster in her responses to simple visual stimuli. Based on these data, normal ammonia levels and lack of overt HE history, she was qualified as free of both HE and other significant neurological and psychiatric diseases. Given that she was being considered for transplantation, brain MRI was prescribed, and found to be normal. At over 1 year, she remains well mentally and her cirrhosis has not decompensated further.

Difficult HE Diagnosis 2: A Patient with High Cognitive Reserve

The concept of cognitive reserve refers to the mental ability to cope with brain damage [8]. Cognitive reserve is related to life-long cognitive stimulation produced by education, working and leisure-time activities, as well as by biological and genetic factors. Cognitive reserve has been proven to influence the cognitive expression of HE [9]. Here we report the case of a high-performing young electronic engineer, who developed profound EEG changes compatible with HE in the complete absence of any degree of cognitive dysfunction. He was 34 years old when he was referred to our unit in 2000 for transplant workup, because of rapidly decompensating HCV-related cirrhosis (Child C13). He had ascites and was jaundiced and malnourished. Plasma ammonia level was 78 µmol/L (<35 µmol/L). In neuropsychological examination he was normal: PHES was +1 with excellent performances on all tests (for example, digit symbol: 56 items in 90 s). His EEG was severely slowed, and dominated by delta-theta activity (Fig. 8.3). On

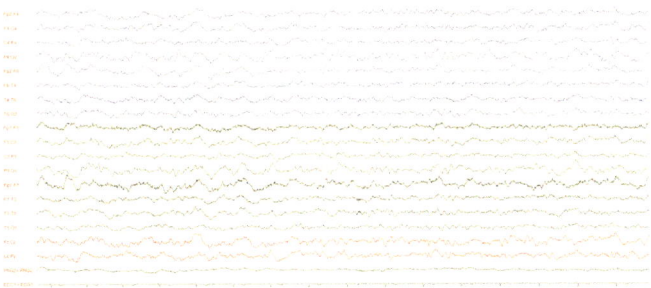

Fig. 8.3 Severely slowed, delta-theta-dominated EEG (longitudinal montage; 20 s; blue = right hemisphere, front to back; black = left hemisphere, front to back, red = central areas)

spectral analysis, the mean frequency was 5.6 Hz, relative delta power 45% and theta relative power 40%, which would be classified as grade III according to the Van der Rijt-Amodio classification [10, 11]. Had this HE phenotype been apparent clinically, he would have met the criteria for the diagnosis of fulminant hepatic failure. He died a few weeks later of a variceal bleeding whilst on the transplant list. In this instance, HE was diagnosed on neurophysiological bases, as the patient's age and cognitive reserve allowed him to compensate very well, virtually abolishing any clinical/cognitive expression of the disease.

Conclusions

According to the joint AASLD-EASL guideline definition [5], HE is a 'brain dysfunction caused by liver insufficiency and/or portal-systemic shunt; it manifests as a wide spectrum of neurological or psychiatric abnormalities ranging from subclinical alterations to coma'. Such definition establishes a clear causal relation between HE and underlying liver insufficiency/shunt, and it does not imply the absence of co-existing neurological disorders. These are crucial aspects of the definition, because HE is unspecific phenotypically, and in real practice several conditions may overlap to impair mental function in patients with cirrhosis/shunt. Also, the clinical expression of HE is modulated by premorbid performance, which is generally difficult to establish when the issue of diagnosing/excluding HE arises. As illustrated by the case histories, when trying to diagnose or exclude HE, it is very useful to:

1. Understand the neuropsychological profile of HE, which is characterized by abnormalities in psychomotor speed, attention and executive function. These tend to arise in a gradual

rather than abrupt fashion, often in relation to well-defined precipitating events.
2. Monitor changes in clinical, cognitive and neurophysiological variables in response to treatment of precipitants and maximal ammonia-lowering treatment, preferably having documented hyperammonaemia in the first place.
3. Institute differential diagnosis algorithms, based on a set of laboratory variables (full blood count, electrolytes, ammonia, TSH, CRP, glycaemia, vitamin B12 and urine analysis [12]) and cerebral imaging.
4. Combine multiple assessment modalities, in line with the original proposal by Conn and colleagues, who developed a simple HE index based on behavioural, cognitive, neurophysiological and biochemical variables [13].

While point 4 may require some specialist experience, points 1–3 are easily applicable in any clinical context, as long as clinicians are clear about (i) the disease definition and (ii) the importance of establishing the pathophysiology of any mental alteration arising in a patient with cirrhosis, and treat it accordingly.

References

1. Pugh RN, Murray-Lyon IM, Dawson JL, Pietroni MC, Williams R. Transection of the oesophagus for bleeding oesophageal varices. Br J Surg. 1973;60:646–9.
2. Kamath PS, Wiesner RH, Malinchoc M, Kremers W, Therneau TM, Kosberg CL, et al. A model to predict survival in patients with end-stage liver disease. Hepatology. 2001;33:464–70.
3. Biggins SW, Kim WR, Terrault NA, Saab S, Balan V, Schiano T, et al. Evidence-based incorporation of serum sodium concentration into MELD. Gastroenterology. 2006;130:1652–60.
4. Folstein MF, Folstein SE, McHugh PR. "Mini-mental state". A practical method for grading the cognitive state of patients for the clinician. J Psychiatr Res. 1975;12:189–98.

5. Vilstrup H, Amodio P, Bajaj J, Cordoba J, Ferenci P, Mullen KD, et al. Hepatic encephalopathy in chronic liver disease: 2014 Practice Guideline by the American Association for the Study of Liver Diseases and the European Association for the Study of the Liver. Hepatology. 2014;60:715–35.
6. Teasdale G, Jennett B. Assessment of coma and impaired consciousness. A practical scale. Lancet. 1974;2:81–4.
7. Weissenborn K, Ennen JC, Schomerus H, Ruckert N, Hecker H. Neuropsychological characterization of hepatic encephalopathy. J Hepatol. 2001;34:768–73.
8. Alexander GE, Furey ML, Grady CL, Pietrini P, Brady DR, Mentis MJ, et al. Association of premorbid intellectual function with cerebral metabolism in Alzheimer's disease: implications for the cognitive reserve hypothesis. Am J Psychiatry. 1997;154:165–72.
9. Van der Rijt CC, Schalm SW, De Groot GH, De Vlieger M. Objective measurement of hepatic encephalopathy by means of automated EEG analysis. Electroencephalogr Clin Neurophysiol. 1984;57:423–6.
10. Amodio P, Montagnese S, Spinelli G, Schiff S, Mapelli D. Cognitive reserve is a resilience factor for cognitive dysfunction in hepatic encephalopathy. Metab Brain Dis. 2017;32:1287–93.
11. Amodio P, Marchetti P, Del Piccolo F, de Tourtchaninoff M, Varghese P, Zuliani C, et al. Spectral versus visual EEG analysis in mild hepatic en-cephalopathy. Clin Neurophysiol. 1999;110:1334–44.
12. Romero-Gómez M, Montagnese S, Jalan R. Hepatic encephalopathy in patients with acute decompensation of cirrhosis and acute-on-chronic liver failure. J Hepatol. 2015;62:437–47.
13. Conn HO, Leevy CM, Vlahcevic ZR, Rodgers JB, Maddrey WC, Seeff L, et al. Comparison of lactulose and neomycin in the treatment of chronic portal-systemic encephalopathy. A double blind controlled trial. Gastroenterology. 1977;72:573–83.

Chapter 9
Integrating Palliative Principles into Cirrhosis Care: The Effect of Hepatic Encephalopathy

Michael Ney, Amanda Brisebois, and Puneeta Tandon

Case 1

Mr. S is a previously healthy 60-year-old man referred to hepatology clinic with a new diagnosis of suspected alcoholic cirrhosis. He has a long history of alcoholism dating back to his early 20s and currently drinks 6–8 alcoholic beverages per day. He does not smoke and has never used illicit drugs. He has no other contributing causes for chronic liver disease. His primary

Amanda Brisebois and Puneeta Tandon contributed equally to this work.

M. Ney, M.D.
Division of Gastroenterology, University of Alberta,
Edmonton, AB, Canada
e-mail: mney@ualberta.ca

A. Brisebois
Division of Palliative Care and General Internal Medicine,
University of Alberta, Edmonton, AB, Canada
e-mail: amandab@ualberta.ca

P. Tandon (✉)
Cirrhosis Care Clinic, Division of Gastroenterology, University of Alberta,
Edmonton, AB, Canada
e-mail: ptandon@ualberta.ca

© Springer International Publishing AG, part of Springer Nature 2018   129
J. S. Bajaj (ed.), *Diagnosis and Management of Hepatic Encephalopathy*, https://doi.org/10.1007/978-3-319-76798-7_9

symptoms include increasing abdominal girth, abdominal pain, leg swelling, fatigue, and jaundice. He reports no overt confusion but has had some difficulty sleeping at night and finds that he requires frequent daytime naps. Due to these symptoms, he has been unable to work for the last month. On physical examination, he has muscle wasting, scleral icterus, and a soft, nontender abdomen with moderate ascites and bilateral pedal edema. He is oriented to person, place, and time and does not have asterixis. On his workup, his liver enzymes are just above the upper limit of normal and he has abnormal liver function (total bilirubin 55 µmol/L, INR 1.9, albumin 27 g/L), sodium 132 mmol/L, and creatinine 78 µmol/L with platelets of 90 ($\times 10^9$/L). His Na-MELD is 22. His abdominal ultrasound confirms a cirrhotic appearing liver, splenomegaly, and moderate ascites with no evidence of hepatocellular carcinoma (HCC).

Mr. S is counseled as to the etiology of his liver disease as well as the severity. It is made clear that he would not be eligible for liver transplantation unless he completes an alcohol rehabilitation program and abstinence requirements. Arrangements are made for him to see a dietician to discuss a low-salt and high-protein and -calorie diet. He is given a prescription for furosemide and spironolactone for ascites/edema management and is given a routine blood work requisition. He is booked for a gastroscopy to screen for varices. Ultrasounds are arranged on a 6-monthly basis to screen for HCC. He is scheduled for a follow-up appointment in clinic in 3 months' time for reassessment.

Unfortunately, over the next month Mr. S continues to drink alcohol and is admitted to the hospital 1 month after his initial assessment with hepatic encephalopathy (HE). He has been constipated at home according to his wife and this, in conjunction with his continued alcohol use, is considered to be the exacerbating factor for his acute HE presentation. He has no evidence of infection or other HE precipitants. He is started on lactulose and his level of consciousness does not improve. Rifaximin is added with partial improvement. His family is upset and confused about his continued deterioration. He continues to decompensate in hospital with the new development of spontaneous bacterial peritonitis and hepatorenal syndrome (HRS). The clinical team initiates advance care planning (ACP) discussions with the family as the patient is too confused to participate in the conversation. It takes a significant effort for the family to understand why he is not a transplant or an intensive care unit candidate and eventually they agree that the focus of care should be compassionate/comfort care. Over the coming days, Mr. S develops severe abdominal pain and leg cramps. Infection is ruled out but his care team is hesitant to prescribe him with anything stronger than acetaminophen to manage his pain. His renal dysfunction progresses and 3 weeks after he is admitted to hospital Mr. S passes away with his family at his side.

Section 1a: Integrating Palliative Principles into General Care of Patients with Cirrhosis—What Are They and Why Are They Important?

The case above will be familiar to practitioners who manage end-stage liver disease. Although at first glance it may seem to have been managed quite well by the physicians involved, there are aspects of the case which highlight the need for a more effective initial assessment and for the early involvement of care with palliative principles. This includes the integration of early ACP discussions as well as screening and management of symptoms including pain.

As defined by the World Health Organization, palliative care is "the active total care of patients whose disease is not responsive to curative treatment." An approach to care using palliative principles improves "the quality of life of patients and their families facing problems associated with life-threatening illness, through the prevention and relief of suffering by means of early identification and impeccable assessment and treatment of pain and other problems, physical, psychosocial and spiritual" [1, 2]. In addition to symptom management, ACP is a central component of care using palliative principles. ACP is defined as a *process* that supports adults at any age or stage of health in understanding and sharing their personal values, life goals, and preferences regarding future medical care [3]. This integrated approach to care has already demonstrated significant benefits in other chronic disease populations including chronic kidney disease, congestive heart failure, chronic obstructive pulmonary disease, and dementia [4–6]. These include improved patients' symptoms, a higher likelihood of dying at home, more focused ACP, better psychosocial health, reduced healthcare utilization, and higher patient/family satisfaction. Data in cirrhosis is limited. In a recent study of delisted liver-transplant candidates [7], the integration of routine palliative care consultation was associated with a shorter duration to "do not resuscitate" (DNR) status, a decrease in ICU stay time, and a positive family response to the incorporation of palliative care consults [7]. Importantly, patient mortality was not hastened by this intervention. Palliative care has also been shown to improve health-related quality of life (HRQoL) and decrease healthcare utilization in cirrhosis [8].

Despite emerging data for the utility of palliative principles in cirrhosis and their well-established role in other end-stage chronic illnesses and cancer, rates of palliative care consultation are low. Recent studies have reported palliative care consultation in 11% of patients ineligible for transplantation [9, 10], with 90% of referrals taking place within 72 h of death [10]. As demonstrated by the case of Mr. S, palliative principles such as early ACP and aggressive symptom control remain underutilized in patients with cirrhosis. There are several recognized barriers that contribute to this underutilization. Prognostication and prediction of the time course of death and disease trajectory are challenging in these patients [11]. Patients with more compensated or well-controlled cirrhosis may not appear as ill as they really are and severe decompensation can occur rapidly [12, 13]. Few clinicians routinely screen for symptoms such as pain or muscle cramps in clinical practice, or feel comfortable managing these symptoms in the setting of cirrhosis. This leads to underestimation of symptom burden and undertreatment [14]. Recent reviews of cirrhosis do not include symptom management in their algorithms [15–17]. Lastly, there is a common misconception about the role of palliative care as being limited to the last few days of life [18]. It is vital to remember that palliative care is not simply about quelling the inevitable tide of death, but more importantly hinges upon enriching the patient life that yet remains. Palliative principles are applicable to patients with years of life still left to live, but with serious illness and high symptom burden.

While it has been suggested that specific symptoms of decompensated liver disease, such as ascites or HE, could be used as potential triggers for a palliative care consult [19], ideally, palliative care principles and end-of-life planning should be instituted in some capacity in all patients with cirrhosis and certainly prior to the onset of HE. This early integration of ACP can be applied by all healthcare practitioners and does not require consultation from trained palliative care health practitioners who may be needed in more severe cases or at the end of life.

Section 1b: Palliative Principles as They Apply to Hepatic Encephalopathy

Existing HE guidelines published by the American Association for the Study of the Liver Diseases (AASLD) and the European Association for the Study of the Liver (EASL) have not been expanded to cover palliative care, symptom-focused care, effect on a patient's psychosocial and spiritual needs, or suggestions

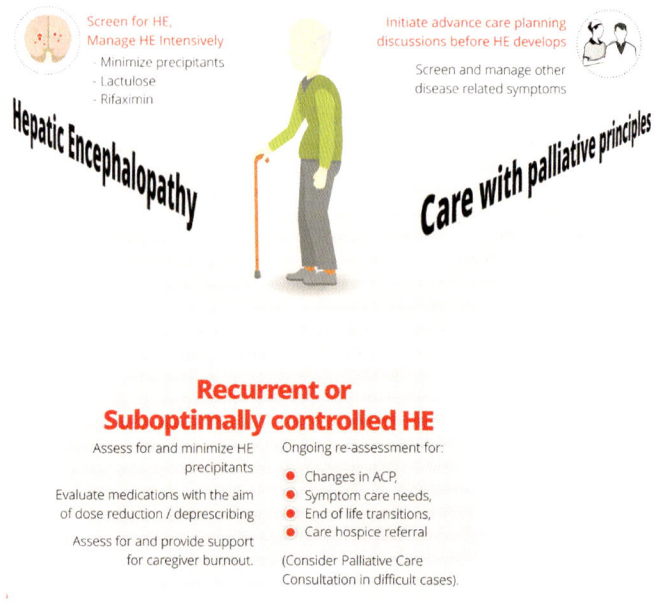

Fig. 9.1 The common road between hepatic encephalopathy management and care with palliative principles

for when palliative care involvement should be sought [20]. Several intersection points are seen between palliative principles and HE including the management of HE itself as a debilitating symptom of the disease, the effect that HE has on the ability to carry out ACP discussions (Fig. 9.1), the effect that other medications may have on precipitating HE (Case 2), and lastly the impact of HE on the caregiver (Case 3).

Overt HE is common in the final months of life for patients with cirrhosis (8% prevalence in the final 3–6 months and 31% prevalence in the final month) [21]. It has a major impact on HRQoL, employability, driving ability, and personal independence [22, 23]. Even minimal HE (MHE), which requires specialized neurocognitive testing to diagnose, has been associated with decreased HRQoL, reduced cognitive function, sleep disturbance, driving impairment, falls, and increased mortality [24]. The medical management of HE in the last months of life is similar to the general management of HE, and typically falls in the hands of the non-palliative care specialist (e.g., gastroenterology, general internal medicine). Lactulose is the mainstay of therapy but where necessary rifaximin can be a useful addition when HE is refractory to lactulose or if patients are unable to tolerate lactulose [20, 25]. Other therapies with less well-established evidence such as branched-chain amino acids (BCAAs), metabolic ammonia scavengers, L-ornithine L-aspartate (LOLA), probiotics, glutaminase inhibitors, neomycin, metronidazole, and flumazenil can be considered on a case-by-case basis, especially in the setting of refractory HE, and are beyond the scope of this chapter [20].

HE is a major factor that impacts a patient's ability to effectively engage in ACP discussions [26]. This highlights the importance of early ACP, and the relevance of a surrogate decision maker [3, 27, 28]. In addition to being an extra set of ears to recall information once out of the clinic, surrogates can help the patient to understand the ACP process. In circumstances where the patient has HE and is unable to make their own decisions about their care, a surrogate works "with clinicians to make the best possible in-the-moment medical decisions" based on the patient's values, goals, and preferences [29, 30].

In the case of Mr. S, palliative principles could have been applied from initial consultation (ACP discussion regarding the importance of symptom control as well as the possible complications of cirrhosis). This was of particular relevance given his history of day-night reversal, suggesting HE. A preliminary ACP discussion would have allowed Mr. S time to consider his wishes for care should his health deteriorate and reduce future stress on the family in making difficult judgments without his input. Lastly, appropriate pain control in his final few days of life could have had a significant impact on his overall HRQoL. We find that with appropriate education, symptom management and early ACP can be broached by primary specialists. Palliative practitioners can offer additional assistance with more challenging symptom management issues, address difficult end-of-life issues and caregiver discord, and provide information on available hospital and community resources. Although not all patients will wish for this type of detailed information, even in cases where they do not, caregivers may benefit from the information to help with planning and the coping process.

Case 2

Mrs. P is a 66-year-old lady with a long-standing diagnosis of nonalcoholic steatohepatitis (NASH) cirrhosis, currently admitted for symptom management in the setting of refractory ascites and poorly controlled HE. She has a past medical history significant for morbid obesity, type II diabetes, coronary artery disease, osteoporosis, and osteoarthritis. She is currently not listed for liver transplantation due to her severe obesity and poor control of her medical comorbidities. Her HE had been managed effectively as an outpatient with lactulose up until her current admission to hospital. A week prior, she was admitted with spontaneous bacterial peritonitis (SBP) and HE. Since admission, she has improved with the addition of rifaximin to her lactulose therapy and treatment of her SBP with a third-generation cephalosporin. She is requiring weekly paracenteses in hospital for refractory ascites and is not felt to be a candidate for transjugular intrahepatic portosystemic shunt (TIPS) in the setting of her history of HE.

Mrs. P describes constant pain in her joints, lower back, and abdomen. In addition, she has difficulty sleeping and her family thinks she may be depressed. Mrs. P and her family ask what else might be done to better manage her pain and insomnia. The team is concerned about starting any medications that might exacerbate her HE. A resident on the team suggests a palliative care consult.

Section 2: Hepatic Encephalopathy and Medication Management—Choosing Wisely and De-prescribing

HE can be exacerbated by all of the classic precipitants discussed in previous chapters. Specifically, many of the drugs commonly used for symptom control are known precipitants of HE (opioids, antidepressants, anxiolytics, neuroleptics, and benzodiazepines). Constipation and dehydration are more common symptoms in patients with end-organ failure [31, 32], and can affect medication metabolism and elimination. In cirrhosis, a balance needs to be struck between patient comfort and risk of progressive HE. This requires an understanding of medication metabolism, combined with a cautious approach to prescribing.

Cirrhosis is associated with decreased hepatic blood flow and shunting which leads to slower metabolism of drugs processed by the liver and resulting increased bioavailability of many medications [33]. Other complicating factors include a relatively decreased serum albumin in most patients, and changes in body water stores, leading to an altered volume of distribution [33].

Accordingly, the avoidance of nonessential medications is vital and a non-pharmacological focus of symptom management should be sought wherever possible. Although evolving, literature is sparse when assessing the potential utility of non-pharmacological interventions, even in more well-studied areas such as pain management in cancer patients [34]. Interventions such as transcutaneous electrical nerve stimulation, massage, exercise, cognitive therapy, acupuncture, biofeedback, and reflexology have been investigated with mixed results in cancer patients for pain management [34]. Overall, evidence for these interventions is moderate in cancer and nonexistent in the cirrhosis literature, but their low-risk nature in comparison to more aggressive pharmacological options warrants their consideration as a first-line option.

Medication Adjustments Necessary in Liver Dysfunction: Symptom Management

It is beyond the scope of this review to provide an exhaustive review of the literature in this area. We provide some practical tips for medication adjustments that may be necessary to reduce the risk of HE for common symptoms (Table 9.1). Relevant, more in-depth reviews in the area are referenced.

Table 9.1 Recommendations for the use of common palliative care medications in the setting of cirrhosis and HE

Medication or medication class	Recommended dosing
Fentanyl	No dosing change
	Use minimum dose possible due to risk of HE
Remifentanil	No dosing change
	Use minimum dose possible due to risk of HE
Morphine, hydromorphone, oxycodone	Dose reduction required (suggest 50%) and decrease dosing frequency
	Use minimum dose possible due to risk of HE
	Extreme care in HRS

Table 9.1 (continued)

Medication or medication class	Recommended dosing
Tramadol	Avoid. Can accumulate, consider alternatives
Codeine	Cautious dosing on a case-by-case basis (may be ineffective for some patients as metabolized to morphine in the liver)
Gabapentin, pregabalin (calcium channel ligands)	Unaltered. No dosing change. First line for neuropathic pain
Dextropropoxyphene	Avoid
Pethidine/meperidine	Avoid
Acetaminophen/paracetamol	Maximum 2 g per day
NSAIDs	Avoid
Benzodiazepines	Avoid or utilize at very small doses watching for HE exacerbation
SNRIs	Dose reduction required E.g. Mirtazapine—clearance reduced by 30% Venlafaxine—reduce dose by 50% Duloxetine—avoid due to liver toxicity
TCAs	Dose reduction required Nortriptyline and desipramine likely preferable to others, watch for significant side effects (anticholinergic)
SSRIs	E.g., Sertraline Slowly up-titrate to a targeted maximal dose of 50% normal
Antihistamine	Hydroxyzine—25 mg at bedtime (12.5 mg if history of HE, TIPS, or age >65)

(continued)

Table 9.1 (continued)

Medication or medication class	Recommended dosing
Antiemetics	Dimenhydrinate—avoid, too sedating
	Metoclopramide—no dose adjustment
	Ondansetron—no dose adjustment
	Child-Pugh A/B
	—8 mg/day max dose Child-Pugh C
Antianxiety, antiemetic	Haldol—no dose reduction required, decreases seizure threshold, therefore use with caution in patients at risk for withdrawal seizures
	Olanzapine—progressively sedating, use at lowest possible dose

Pain

Acetaminophen/paracetamol is the preferred form of analgesia for patients with cirrhosis, especially where there is an increased concern for HE. The maximum recommended daily dose is 2 g as its half-life is nearly doubled in severe liver failure [35]. While acetaminophen/paracetamol is not always effective for more severe pain, it is a good first step in the palliative pain management of patients with cirrhosis. Nonsteroidal anti-inflammatory drugs (NSAIDs) are associated with varying degrees of hepatic clearance. ASA and ibuprofen elimination is unchanged in liver disease. Naproxen has a markedly reduced elimination (about 60%) [36]. While NSAIDs are not known to increase the risk of HE, due to their well-established adverse effects, these medications are not recommended in patients with cirrhosis [37]. Gabapentin and pregabalin do not accumulate in cirrhosis and are reasonable first-line options for neuropathic pain [38, 39].

Opioids are commonly used for the management of pain in the palliative care setting, but as previously mentioned they can increase the risk of HE due to their neuromodulatory effects and also due to the constipation they induce [40, 41]. The liver is the primary site of metabolism for the majority of opioids via the CYP2D6 and 3A4 oxidation pathways or via glucuronidation [42]. While glucuronidation is less affected in patients with cirrhosis, the CYP system is deranged in liver disease and is also affected by malnutrition and altered protein intake [43]. In our experience, if users are aware of the limitations and follow the principle of starting with very low dosing and up-titrating slowly [44], in most cases opioids can be used effectively and safely. It remains unclear which opioid is best for use in cirrhosis. Although fentanyl is not metabolized via the liver [45, 46], it can be difficult to administer and titrate, limiting its use. Both morphine and hydromorphone (including the extended-release formulations) can be used but require dose reductions due to moderately impaired clearance [37, 47–50]. Oxycodone has severely impaired elimination and therefore ideally should be completely avoided or dosing significantly reduced [51]. Tramadol and codeine are both activated in the liver and are less effective in cirrhosis. Dextropropoxyphene and pethidine/meperidine should be avoided due to the potential for liver toxicity and an increased risk of seizures in patients with HE, respectively [36, 44]. The options for opioid-based therapy in the setting of hepatorenal syndrome (HRS) are very limited as morphine, hydromorphone, and pethidine/meperidine all have varying degrees of renal clearance [52].

Anxiety and Depression

Benzodiazepines are commonly used for the treatment of anxiety. Although cirrhosis does not have a significant influence on the metabolism of medications such as lorazepam, temazepam, and to a lesser extent oxazepam, the risk of HE with benzodiazepines in general is too high to justify their use [53–56]. When treatment is required for agitation in palliative patients with HE, haldol is our initial choice, although care needs to be taken in patients at risk of seizures (such as alcohol withdrawal) as it decreases the seizure threshold [57, 58].

Antidepressants of different classes have diverse pharmaco-kinetic profiles in cirrhosis. Serotonin and norepinephrine uptake inhibitors (SNRIs) like venlafaxine and duloxetine have moderate-to-severe impaired clearance in cirrhosis. Venlafaxine dosing should be adjusted accordingly and duloxetine should be avoided entirely due to risks of hepatotoxicity [59, 60]. For tri-cyclic antidepressants (TCAs), accumulation is likely, with increased plasma levels of amitriptyline in patients with cirrho-sis [61]. Nortriptyline and desipramine are likely preferable to amitriptyline and imipramine as they are equally efficacious and are less sedating [52]. If used, practitioners should watch for side effects that particularly affect patients with risk of HE, such as constipation [39]. Selective serotonin reuptake inhibi-tors (SSRIs) are likely to be the safest antidepressant options in cirrhosis [62]. All SSRIs have reduced clearance in cirrhosis with citalopram lowest at a 36% reduction and sertraline highest at a 70% reduction [62–64]. SSRIs should be routinely pre-scribed to target a 50% lower maximum dose, with slow up-titration and careful monitoring in a palliative cirrhosis population [62]. Finally, antiemetics are not known to precipi-tate HE so they can be used where required to palliate patients with cirrhosis, although dimenhydrinate should ideally be avoided due to its sedative effects.

Sleep and Other Factors

Sleep difficulties are challenging to manage in patients at risk for HE. First-line therapy should involve attempts to control HE, as HE in itself can lead to sleep dysfunction. The H1 recep-tor blocker hydroxyzine has demonstrated benefit in improving sleep in patients with cirrhosis, although it did precipitate overt HE in 1 of 35 patients studied with MHE. A dose of 25 mg at bedtime was prescribed and this dose was decreased to 12.5 mg in those with a history of overt HE, TIPS, or age >65 [65]. While trial data is otherwise limited on etiological treatments for sleep disturbance in cirrhosis, sleep and light hygiene practices should be encouraged and caution should be taken with all hypnotics due to their inherent risk of precipitating HE [66].

Measures to avoid other HE risk factors such as dehydration, SBP, and constipation should be taken in all patients. Although they have no major change in their pharmacokinetics in cirrhosis, diuretics such as spironolactone and furosemide should be used judiciously in the patient with advanced cirrhosis, balancing patient comfort in the alleviation of ascites and pedal edema, with the potential for dehydration and HE exacerbation [67, 68]. Prophylaxis for SBP with antibiotics such as norfloxacin should be continued to decrease the risk of secondary HE. As previously alluded to, caution should be taken to avoid constipation via traditional means (such as PEG 3350 and lactulose).

De-prescribing in Cirrhosis: Critical Component to Consider to Limit HE at the End of Life

Little literature exists to guide practitioners on downscaling medications as cirrhosis progresses and patient function and quality of life decline. In keeping with general palliative principles, an attempt should be made to limit nonessential medications in the final weeks and days of life. Common medications that may be discontinued in the palliative setting include statins, antihypertensive medications, hypoglycemic agents, bisphosphonates, and antidementia drugs [69]. Symptomatic control is paramount in the final stages of disease and this should be the focus of care. Medical therapies align with the goals outlined by the patient and family via ACP. In the final days of life, it is accepted that confusion may be prevalent, and that the emphasis for treatment shifts to ameliorating pain, dyspnea, anxiety, and other troublesome symptoms as opposed to complete HE/super-imposed delirium clearance. In the final hours of life, a complete cessation of the patient's regular medications may be necessary and palliative sedation may be required in order to best serve the dying patient [70].

Consulting Palliative Care to Aid in Therapeutic Decisions

For our case, a palliative care consult is appropriate. Not only will this provide assistance with end-of-life management, but symptomatic management as well, the primary challenge for Mrs. P. Antiemetics should be trialed for her, metoclopramide being a good starting medication. Haloperidol may also be considered if unsuccessful or agitation is also a predominant concern. She can be started on acetaminophen to a maximum dose of 2 g/day and if this is not sufficient the cautious use of an opioid such as hydromorphone would be a reasonable option to trial for her pain. In consultation with palliative care, a psychiatry consult may also be necessary to determine the utility of starting a low-dose SSRI such as citalopram, targeting a maximal dose of 50% of that which would be typically prescribed.

Case3

Mr. K is a 53-year-old man with Child-Pugh C alcoholic cirrhosis who comes to clinic with his wife for routine follow-up. He has been abstinent from alcohol for 2 years and is on the liver transplant wait-list. His major concern is of worsening ascites, which is partially controlled with increasing doses of furosemide and spironolactone. Otherwise, he has been feeling "okay," with no overt confusion or GI bleeding. His most recent abdominal ultrasound reveals no evidence of HCC. Mr. K is referred for therapeutic paracenteses on an as-needed basis. Prior to the end of the appointment, Mrs. K expresses some concerns that Mr. K has been feeling "down" lately. She has been finding it increasingly stressful to care for him as she finds that he is less able to participate in his care and has trouble following directions. She is reassured by the hepatologist that better control of Mr. K's ascites should help the situation and a suggestion is made encouraging her to follow up with her family physician in regard to her own mental well-being.

Three months later, Mr. and Mrs. K are back for another follow-up appointment. Mr. K now appears overtly confused on exam and asterixis is present. Mrs. K is clearly quite distraught, noting that her husband has been intermittently confused like this over the past couple of months and she can no longer cope with this. She doesn't understand why this is happening and isn't sure that she can go on at home any longer with her husband's escalating care needs. She can no longer work and thus money is becoming increasingly tight. She begins to cry, and asks "is there anything you can do to help us?"

Section 3: How Hepatic Encephalopathy Affects Caregivers—The Palliative Principle of Psychosocial and Spiritual Needs

Informal caregivers are an essential component of the medical management of chronically ill patients and are vital to the financial viability of North American health care [71, 72]. Although not studied directly in cirrhosis, patient outcomes improve with the involvement of informal caregivers [73]. Their involvement leads to less complications and fewer hospital admissions [74–

77]. Informal caregivers are responsible for much of the care provided to patients with cirrhosis, taking a major role in medication management and administration of palliative care [75]. In their 2012 study, Rakoski et al. found that one-third of patients with cirrhosis identified an informal caregiver [75]. These patients required twice the number of informal caregiving hours per week when compared to an age-matched population.

The responsibility of caring for an ill relative or friend can be physically and emotionally taxing, with studies showing increased rates of depression [78], worse HRQoL [79], and overall health [80] and even increased mortality in caregivers [81]. Like other chronic illnesses, many caregivers for patients with cirrhosis experience caregiver burden [82]. Risk factors for a more severe perceived caregiver burden in cirrhosis include HE [82, 83], female gender of caregiver [84], alcoholic etiology of cirrhosis [85], and a higher model for end-stage liver disease (MELD) score [85]. Caregiver burden in the setting of cirrhosis has deleterious effects on HRQoL [86, 87], psychosocial functioning [86, 87], family finances [21], and personal mental health and vitality for the caregiver [87]. In their 2016 study, Kunzler-Heule et al. also found that caregivers in cirrhosis reported more responsibility for day-to-day activities such as housework, alterations in their other personal relationships, and feeling tied down to their partners in that they could not leave them alone without fear of negative consequences [88]. All of these factors may contribute to caregiver burnout. Moreover, it is recognized that many caregivers have limited social support [82], further exacerbating the risk for these individuals.

Importantly, the degree of neuropsychiatric impairment displayed by patients with cirrhosis correlates with worsening caregiver burnout and has a greater affect on caregiver schedules, sense of entrapment, and self-assessed personal health [82, 83]. A more substantial HE burden predisposes to greater patient unemployment and a worse financial status [82, 83], which of course impact the finances of the entire family unit. Kunzler-Heule et al. specifically analyzed 12 caregivers of patients with cirrhosis and found that HE had a severe impact on their lives [88]. Five different themes were identified by these family members including feeling overwhelmed by the unexplained symptoms and behaviors of the patient, learning after the fact that these behaviors were secondary to HE, learning the symptoms of HE, feelings of being tied down, and finally overcoming obstacles to working with healthcare providers. In keeping with this, data from other studies support that although informal caregivers serve a crucial role in patient care, they often feel undertrained, underprepared, and a lack of support/acknowledgement from healthcare providers for the services they provide [74, 89].

What can be done to impact caregiver burnout? Ideally, caregivers should be proactively incorporated into the healthcare and palliation plan and provided with education about HE, how to avoid precipitants, its presentation, and its therapy [88]. A greater degree of awareness of HE and its treatment is associated with a better HRQoL [83]. In keeping with Case 1, ACP should be incorporated as early as possible, ideally prior to the onset of HE. This may prevent the caregiver and family from making uncomfortable decisions without full input from their loved one as the disease progresses.

Caregiver stress may be considered a trigger for palliative care consultation. Specialized palliative care services have been associated with both short- and long-term caregiver outcomes [90]. Although not formally investigated in the setting of cirrhosis and HE, other strategies for easing caregiver burden are becoming more well established and should be trialed in patients with cirrhosis. Potential interventions include multidisciplinary care with a social worker and a psychologist as well as focused family psychoeducation [74, 91]. Targeted interventions to increase caregiver effectiveness, such as telephone interventions and caregiver support groups, have been effective in other populations [92–94] and may also prove to be of benefit in HE. A short program of mindfulness and supportive group therapy proved beneficial for the management of caregiver burden in a recent study in patients with cirrhosis [95].

At some point, patients with cirrhosis may become too sick to live at home any longer. This can be due to substantial care needs, caregiver burnout, and exhaustion of external assistance such as home care. If not already involved, the palliative care team can provide much-needed assistance in navigating these tumultuous end-of-life issues. While it is easier to consider hospice in patients who are not candidates for transplantation, recent evidence has suggested that hospice may also benefit patients awaiting a potential liver transplant [19, 96]. Hospice is currently underutilized by patients with cirrhosis. Data from the US National Hospice and Palliative Care Organization cite cirrhosis as the fifth most common non-cancer diagnosis to result in hospice care with a diagnosis of cirrhosis in only less than 2% of all hospice patients [97]. The late initiation of hospice care can lead to further reductions in HRQoL [98] and higher healthcare spending [99]. Unfortunately, we lack comprehensive guidelines to assist practitioners with appropriate hospice referral [19].

The case of Mr. and Mrs. K, brings up several relevant issues. First is the lack of appropriate medical therapy for his HE, which should have been suspected on his first visit but was clearly identifiable by his second visit. In addition to controlling symptoms and reducing hospitalizations, appropriate therapy is associated with an improved health-related quality of life [20]. Mrs. K, who demonstrated early signs of caregiver burnout at the first appointment, continued to decline by the second appointment. Much of this may have been alleviated if her husband's HE symptoms had been recognized and treated and if measures had been taken to provide caregiver education regarding cirrhosis-associated complications. The circumstances surrounding the initial visit likely should have triggered at minimum a home-care assessment. Input from social work and psychology/psychiatry could have been sought and an attempt to set Mrs. K up with a cirrhosis caregiver support group could have been made. Palliative care consultation directed for Mrs. K would have been reasonable at any point during the case. All of these factors could have helped to alleviate some of the incredible burden experienced by Mrs. K in the setting of her husband's cirrhosis.

Summary

1. Early ACP is of critical importance in patients with cirrhosis, especially due to the risk of recurrent and unpredictable HE.
2. Encourage early selection of a surrogate decision maker, and the legal documentation of such.
3. Ensure a focus on including a patient's surrogate decision maker in early ACP discussions, and understanding patient and family values early in the illness. This will heighten the ability to support the patient and family throughout the disease trajectory, especially when the patient is no longer able to be involved in conversations due to HE.
4. Medication usage modification is important to consider due to the multiple factors affected by liver dysfunction.
5. Ensure that non-pharmacologic treatments are considered first.
6. Adjust medication dosage and selection based on liver metabolism.
7. Initiate de-prescribing in the last months to weeks of life based on prognosis and patient preference.
8. Caregiver burnout is common in HE, is associated with significant reductions in health and HRQoL, and can be an indication for palliative care consultation.

References

1. World Health Organization Definition of Palliative Care. Retrieved from http://www.who.int/cancer/palliative/definition/en/. Accessed on March 19, 2018.
2. Brisebois AJ, Tandon P. Working with palliative care services. Clin Liver Dis. 2015;6:37–40.
3. Sudore RL, Fried TR. Redefining the "planning" in advance care planning: preparing for end-of-life decision making. Ann Intern Med. 2010;153:256–61.
4. Cohen LM, Moss AH, Weisbord SD, et al. Renal palliative care. J Palliat Med. 2006;9:977–92.
5. Schwarz ER, Baraghoush A, Morrissey RP, et al. Pilot study of palliative care consultation in patients with advanced heart failure referred for cardiac transplantation. J Palliat Med. 2012;15:12–5.
6. Singer AE, Goebel JR, Kim YS, et al. Populations and interventions for palliative and end-of-life care: a systematic review. J Palliat Med. 2016;19:995–1008.
7. Lamba S, Murphy P, McVicker S, et al. Changing end-of-life care practice for liver transplant service patients: structured palliative care intervention in the surgical intensive care unit. J Pain Symptom Manag. 2012;44:508–19.
8. Cordoba J, Flavia M, Jacas C, et al. Quality of life and cognitive function in hepatitis C at different stages of liver disease. J Hepatol. 2003;39:231–8.
9. Poonja Z, Brisebois A, van Zanten SV, et al. Patients with cirrhosis and denied liver transplants rarely receive adequate palliative care or appropriate management. Clin Gastroenterol Hepatol. 2014;12:692–8.
10. Kathpalia P, Smith A, Lai JC. Underutilization of palliative care services in the liver transplant population. World J Transplant. 2016;6:594–8.
11. Larson AM. Palliative care for patients with end-stage liver disease. Curr Gastroenterol Rep. 2015;17:440.
12. D'Amico G, Garcia-Tsao G, Pagliaro L. Natural history and prognostic indicators of survival in cirrhosis: a systematic review of 118 studies. J Hepatol. 2006;44:217–31.
13. Jalan R, Gines P, Olson JC, et al. Acute-on chronic liver failure. J Hepatol. 2012;57:1336–48.
14. Abrams GA, Concato J, Fallon MB. Muscle cramps in patients with cirrhosis. Am J Gastroenterol. 1996;91:1363–6.

15. Muir AJ. Understanding the complexities of cirrhosis. Clin Ther. 2015;37:1822–36.
16. James J, Liou IW. Comprehensive care of patients with chronic liver disease. Med Clin North Am. 2015;99:913–33.
17. McPherson S, Lucey MR, Moriarty KJ. Decompensated alcohol related liver disease: acute management. BMJ. 2016;352:i124.
18. Larson AM, Curtis JR. Integrating palliative care for liver transplant candidates: "too well for transplant, too sick for life". JAMA. 2006;295:2168–76.
19. Potosek J, Curry M, Buss M, et al. Integration of palliative care in end-stage liver disease and liver transplantation. J Palliat Med. 2014;17:1271–7.
20. Vilstrup H, Amodio P, Bajaj J, et al. Hepatic encephalopathy in chronic liver disease: 2014 Practice Guideline by the American Association for the Study of Liver Diseases and the European Association for the Study of the Liver. Hepatology. 2014;60:715–35.
21. Roth K, Lynn J, Zhong Z, et al. Dying with end stage liver disease with cirrhosis: insights from SUPPORT. Study to understand prognoses and preferences for outcomes and risks of treatment. J Am Geriatr Soc. 2000;48:S122–30.
22. Schomerus H, Hamster W. Quality of life in cirrhotics with minimal hepatic encephalopathy. Metab Brain Dis. 2001;16:37–41.
23. Shaw J, Bajaj JS. Covert hepatic encephalopathy: can my patient drive? J Clin Gastroenterol. 2017;51:118–26.
24. Agrawal S, Umapathy S, Dhiman RK. Minimal hepatic encephalopathy impairs quality of life. J Clin Exp Hepatol. 2015;5:S42–8.
25. Bass NM, Mullen KD, Sanyal A, et al. Rifaximin treatment in hepatic encephalopathy. N Engl J Med. 2010;362:1071–81.
26. Arguedas MR, DeLawrence TG, BM MG. Influence of hepatic encephalopathy on health-related quality of life in patients with cirrhosis. Dig Dis Sci. 2003;48:1622–6.
27. McMahan RD, Knight SJ, Fried TR, et al. Advance care planning beyond advance directives: perspectives from patients and surrogates. J Pain Symptom Manag. 2013;46:355–65.
28. Lum HD, Sudore RL, Bekelman DB. Advance care planning in the elderly. Med Clin North Am. 2015;99:391–403.
29. Jackson VA, Jacobsen J, Greer JA, et al. The cultivation of prognostic awareness through the provision of early palliative care in the ambulatory setting: a communication guide. J Palliat Med. 2013;16:894–900.
30. van Vliet LM, Lindenberger E, van Weert JC. Communication with older, seriously ill patients. Clin Geriatr Med. 2015;31:219–30.

31. Clark K, Lam LT, Agar M, et al. The impact of opioids, anticholinergic medications and disease progression on the prescription of laxatives in hospitalized palliative care patients: a retrospective analysis. Palliat Med. 2010;24:410–8.
32. Good P, Richard R, Syrmis W, et al. Medically assisted hydration for adult palliative care patients. Cochrane Database Syst Rev. 2014;(4):Cd006273.
33. Garg RK. Anesthetic considerations in patients with hepatic failure. Int Anesthesiol Clin. 2005;43:45–63.
34. Hokka M, Kaakinen P, Polkki T. A systematic review: non-pharmacological interventions in treating pain in patients with advanced cancer. J Adv Nurs. 2014;70:1954–69.
35. Forrest JA, Adriaenssens P, Finlayson ND, et al. Paracetamol metabolism in chronic liver disease. Eur J Clin Pharmacol. 1979;15:427–31.
36. Rhee C, Broadbent AM. Palliation and liver failure: palliative medications dosage guidelines. J Palliat Med. 2007;10:677–85.
37. Imani F, Motavaf M, Safari S, et al. The therapeutic use of analgesics in patients with liver cirrhosis: a literature review and evidence-based recommendations. Hepat Mon. 2014;14:e23539.
38. Amarapurkar DN. Prescribing medications in patients with decompensated liver cirrhosis. Int J Hepatol. 2011;2011:519526.
39. Dwyer JP, Jayasekera C, Nicoll A. Analgesia for the cirrhotic patient: a literature review and recommendations. J Gastroenterol Hepatol. 2014;29:1356–60.
40. Soleimanpour H, Safari S, Shahsavari Nia K, et al. Opioid drugs in patients with liver disease: a systematic review. Hepat Mon. 2016;16:e32636.
41. Khademi H, Kamangar F, Brennan P, et al. Opioid therapy and its side effects: a review. Arch Iran Med. 2016;19:870–6.
42. Verbeeck RK. Pharmacokinetics and dosage adjustment in patients with hepatic dysfunction. Eur J Clin Pharmacol. 2008;64:1147–61.
43. Chandok N, Watt KD. Pain management in the cirrhotic patient: the clinical challenge. Mayo Clin Proc. 2010;85:451–8.
44. Tegeder I, Lotsch J, Geisslinger G. Pharmacokinetics of opioids in liver disease. Clin Pharmacokinet. 1999;37:17–40.
45. Haberer JP, Schoeffler P, Couderc E, et al. Fentanyl pharmacokinetics in anaesthetized patients with cirrhosis. Br J Anaesth. 1982;54:1267–70.
46. Navapurkar VU, Archer S, Gupta SK, et al. Metabolism of remifentanil during liver transplantation. Br J Anaesth. 1998;81(6):881.
47. Crotty B, Watson KJ, Desmond PV, et al. Hepatic extraction of morphine is impaired in cirrhosis. Eur J Clin Pharmacol. 1989;36:501–6.

48. Hasselstrom J, Eriksson S, Persson A, et al. The metabolism and bioavailability of morphine in patients with severe liver cirrhosis. Br J Clin Pharmacol. 1990;29:289–97.

49. Kotb HI, el-Kabsh MY, Emara SE, et al. Pharmacokinetics of controlled release morphine (MST) in patients with liver cirrhosis. Br J Anaesth. 1997;79(6):804.

50. Durnin C, Hind ID, Ghani SP, et al. Pharmacokinetics of oral immediate-release hydromorphone (Dilaudid IR) in subjects with moderate hepatic impairment. Proc West Pharmacol Soc. 2001;44:83–4.

51. Tallgren M, Olkkola KT, Seppala T, et al. Pharmacokinetics and ventilatory effects of oxycodone before and after liver transplantation. Clin Pharmacol Ther. 1997;61:655–61.

52. Bosilkovska M, Walder B, Besson M, et al. Analgesics in patients with hepatic impairment: pharmacology and clinical implications. Drugs. 2012;72:1645–69.

53. Shull HJ, Wilkinson GR, Johnson R, et al. Normal disposition of oxazepam in acute viral hepatitis and cirrhosis. Ann Intern Med. 1976;84:420–5.

54. Kraus JW, Desmond PV, Marshall JP, et al. Effects of aging and liver disease on disposition of lorazepam. Clin Pharmacol Ther. 1978;24:411–9.

55. Ghabrial H, Desmond PV, Watson KJ, et al. The effects of age and chronic liver disease on the elimination of temazepam. Eur J Clin Pharmacol. 1986;30:93–7.

56. Haussinger D, Schliess F. Pathogenetic mechanisms of hepatic encephalopathy. Gut. 2008;57:1156–65.

57. Prabhakar S, Management BR. Management of agitation and convulsions in hepatic encephalopathy. Indian J Gastroenterol. 2003;22(Suppl 2):S54–8.

58. Lewis J, Stine J. Prescribing medications in patients with cirrhosis–a practical guide. Aliment Pharmacol Ther. 2013;37:1132–56.

59. Holliday SM, Benfield P. Venlafaxine. A review of its pharmacology and therapeutic potential in depression. Drugs. 1995;49:280–94.

60. Suri A, Reddy S, Gonzales C, et al. Duloxetine pharmacokinetics in cirrhotics compared with healthy subjects. Int J Clin Pharmacol Ther. 2005;43:78–84.

61. Hrdina PD, Lapierre YD, Koranyi EK. Altered amitriptyline kinetics in a depressed patient with porto-caval anastomosis. Can J Psychiatr. 1985;30:111–3.

62. Mullish BH, Kabir MS, Thursz MR, et al. Review article: depression and the use of antidepressants in patients with chronic liver disease or liver transplantation. Aliment Pharmacol Ther. 2014;40:880–92.

63. Joffe P, Larsen FS, Pedersen V, et al. Single-dose pharmacokinetics of citalopram in patients with moderate renal insufficiency or hepatic cirrhosis compared with healthy subjects. Eur J Clin Pharmacol. 1998;54:237–42.
64. Demolis JL, Angebaud P, Grange JD, et al. Influence of liver cirrhosis on sertraline pharmacokinetics. Br J Clin Pharmacol. 1996;42:394–7.
65. Spahr L, Coeytaux A, Giostra E, et al. Histamine H1 blocker hydroxyzine improves sleep in patients with cirrhosis and minimal hepatic encephalopathy: a randomized controlled pilot trial. Am J Gastroenterol. 2007;102:744–53.
66. Montagnese S, De Pittà C, De Rui M, et al. Sleep-wake abnormalities in patients with cirrhosis. Hepatology. 2014;59:705–12.
67. Verbeeck RK, Patwardhan RV, Villeneuve JP, et al. Furosemide disposition in cirrhosis. Clin Pharmacol Ther. 1982;31:719–25.
68. Abshagen U, Rennekamp H, Luszpinski G. Disposition kinetics of spironolactone in hepatic failure after single doses and prolonged treatment. Eur J Clin Pharmacol. 1977;11:169–76.
69. Oliveira L, Ferreira MO, Rola A, et al. Deprescription in advanced cancer patients referred to palliative care. J Pain Palliat Care Pharmacother. 2016;30:201–5.
70. Maltoni M, Scarpi E, Rosati M, et al. Palliative sedation in end-of-life care and survival: a systematic review. J Clin Oncol. 2012;30:1378–83.
71. Chari AV, Engberg J, Ray KN, et al. The opportunity costs of informal elder-care in the United States: new estimates from the American Time Use Survey. Health Serv Res. 2015;50:871–82.
72. Hollander MJ, Liu G, Chappell NL. Who cares and how much? The imputed economic contribution to the Canadian healthcare system of middle-aged and older unpaid caregivers providing care to the elderly. Healthc Q. 2009;12:42–9.
73. Smith CE, Piamjariyakul U, Yadrich DM, et al. Complex home care: part III—economic impact on family caregiver quality of life and patients' clinical outcomes. Nurs Econ. 2010;28:393–9. 414
74. Adelman RD, Tmanova LL, Delgado D, et al. Caregiver burden: a clinical review. JAMA. 2014;311:1052–60.
75. Rakoski MO, McCammon RJ, Piette JD, et al. Burden of cirrhosis on older Americans and their families: analysis of the health and retirement study. Hepatology. 2012;55:184–91.
76. Golics CJ, Basra MK, Salek MS, et al. The impact of patients' chronic disease on family quality of life: an experience from 26 specialties. Int J Gen Med. 2013;6:787–98.

77. Jeffs L, Dhalla I, Cardoso R, et al. The perspectives of patients, family members and healthcare professionals on readmissions: preventable or inevitable? J Interprof Care. 2014;28:507–12.

78. Cameron JI, Chu LM, Matte A, et al. One-year outcomes in caregivers of critically ill patients. N Engl J Med. 2016;374:1831–41.

79. Morimoto T, Schreiner AS, Asano H. Caregiver burden and health-related quality of life among Japanese stroke caregivers. Age Ageing. 2003;32:218–23.

80. Pinquart M, Sörensen S. Correlates of physical health of informal caregivers: a meta-analysis. J Gerontol Ser B Psychol Sci Soc Sci. 2007;62:P126–37.

81. Schulz R, Beach SR. Caregiving as a risk factor for mortality: the Caregiver Health Effects Study. JAMA. 1999;282:2215–9.

82. Bajaj JS, Wade JB, Gibson DP, et al. The multi-dimensional burden of cirrhosis and hepatic encephalopathy on patients and caregivers. Am J Gastroenterol. 2011;106:1646–53.

83. Montagnese S, Amato E, Schiff S, et al. A patients' and caregivers' perspective on hepatic encephalopathy. Metab Brain Dis. 2012;27:567–72.

84. Cohen M, Katz D, Baruch Y. Stress among the family caregivers of liver transplant recipients. Prog Transplant. 2007;17:48–53.

85. Miyazaki ET, Dos Santos R Jr, Miyazaki MC, et al. Patients on the waiting list for liver transplantation: caregiver burden and stress. Liver Transpl. 2010;16:1164–8.

86. Rodrigue JR, Dimitri N, Reed A, et al. Quality of life and psychosocial functioning of spouse/partner caregivers before and after liver transplantation. Clin Transpl. 2011;25:239–47.

87. Nguyen DL, Chao D, Ma G, et al. Quality of life and factors predictive of burden among primary caregivers of chronic liver disease patients. Ann Gastroenterol. 2015;28:124–9.

88. Kunzler-Heule P, Beckmann S, Mahrer-Imhof R, et al. Being an informal caregiver for a relative with liver cirrhosis and overt hepatic encephalopathy: a phenomenological study. J Clin Nurs. 2016;25:2559–68.

89. Hasselkus BR, Murray BJ. Everyday occupation, well-being, and identity: the experience of caregivers in families with dementia. Am J Occup Ther. 2007;61:9–20.

90. Abernethy AP, Currow DC, Fazekas BS, et al. Specialized palliative care services are associated with improved short-and long-term caregiver outcomes. Support Care Cancer. 2008;16:585–97.

91. Madigan K, Egan P, Brennan D, et al. A randomised controlled trial of carer-focussed multi-family group psychoeducation in bipolar disorder. Eur Psychiatry. 2012;27(4):281.

92. Hepburn K, Lewis M, Tornatore J, et al. The Savvy Caregiver program: the demonstrated effectiveness of a transportable dementia caregiver psychoeducation program. J Gerontol Nurs. 2007;33:30–6.

93. Grant JS, Elliott TR, Weaver M, et al. Telephone intervention with family caregivers of stroke survivors after rehabilitation. Stroke. 2002;33:2060–5.

94. Chien LY, Chu H, Guo JL, et al. Caregiver support groups in patients with dementia: a meta-analysis. Int J Geriatr Psychiatry. 2011;26:1089–98.

95. Bajaj JS, Ellwood M, Ainger T, et al. Mindfulness-based stress reduction therapy improves patient and caregiver-reported outcomes in cirrhosis. Clin Transl Gastroenterol. 2017;8:e108.

96. Medici V, Rossaro L, Wegelin JA, et al. The utility of the model for end-stage liver disease score: a reliable guide for liver transplant candidacy and, for select patients, simultaneous hospice referral. Liver Transpl. 2008;14:1100–6.

97. Organization NHaPC. NHPCO's facts and figures: hospice care in America; 2015.

98. Christakis NA, Escarce JJ. Survival of Medicare patients after enrollment in hospice programs. N Engl J Med. 1996;335:172–8.

99. Fukui N, Golabi P, Otgonsuren M, et al. Demographics, resource utilization, and outcomes of elderly patients with chronic liver disease receiving hospice care in the United States. Am J Gastroenterol. 2017;112:1700–8.

Index

© Springer International Publishing AG, part of Springer Nature 2018   157
J. S. Bajaj (ed.), *Diagnosis and Management of Hepatic
Encephalopathy*, https://doi.org/10.1007/978-3-319-76798-7

Printed by Printforce, the Netherlands